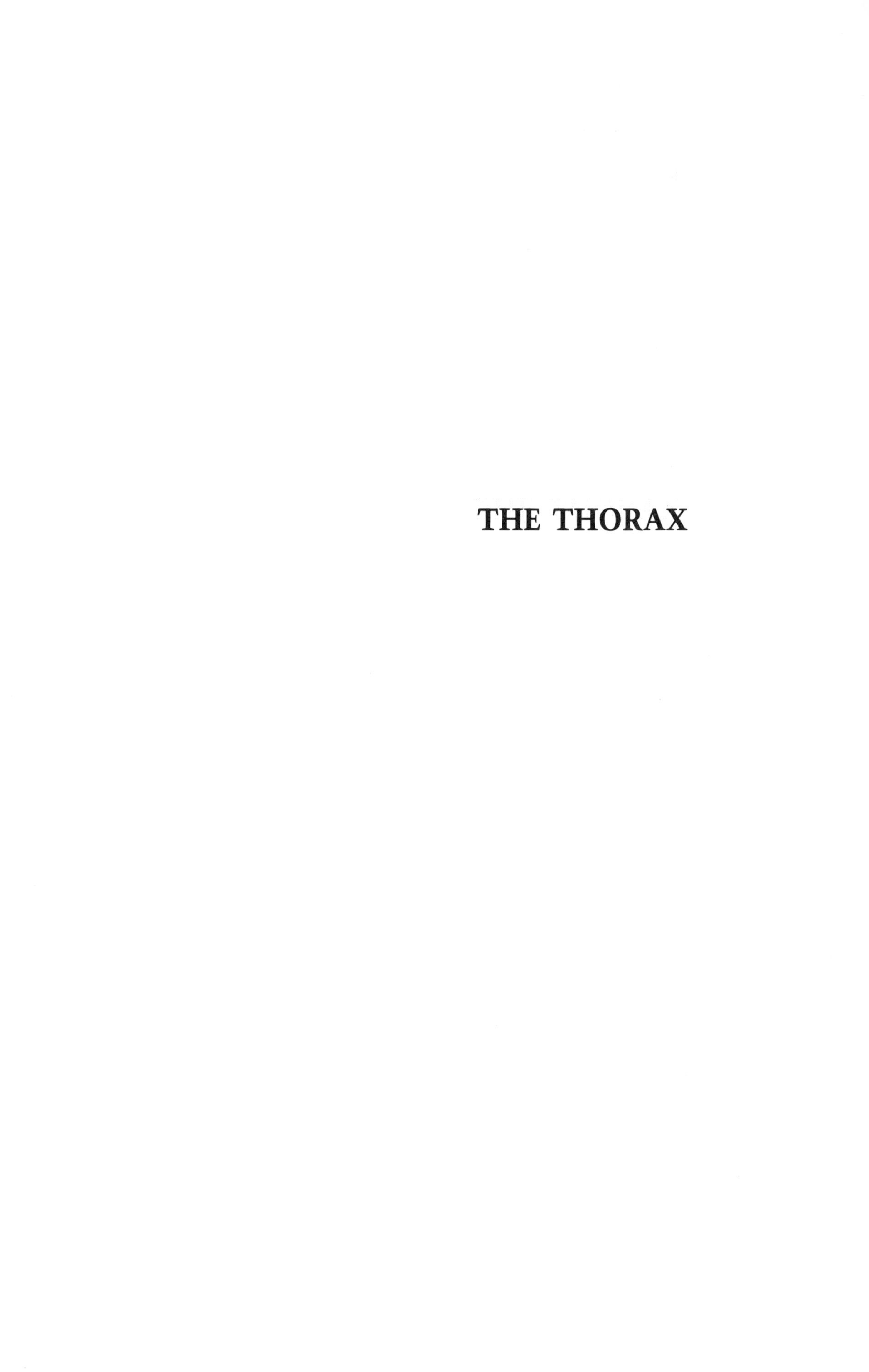

THE THORAX

The Thorax

Jean-Pierre Barral

ILLUSTRATIONS BY
Jacques Roth

Eastland Press
SEATTLE

Originally published as *Le Thorax*
Maloine (Paris), 1989.

P.O. Box 99749, Seattle, Washington, 98139, USA
www.eastlandpress.com

Library of Congress Catalog Card Number: 90-85570
International Standard Book Number: 0-939616-12-2
Printed in the United States of America.

Edited by Daniel Bensky, D.O. and Stephen Anderson, Ph.D. (English edition).
Book design by Gary Niemeier & Catherine L. Nelson

Eighth Printing, 2012

Table of Contents

Introduction

The thorax has two conflicting roles: it must protect the organs enclosed within it while also allowing exchanges with other body cavities. These exchanges occur according to differences in intracavitary pressures and to satisfactory harmony between the tissues which make up the cavities. We think of the vital organs as being protected by the rigidity of the thorax; in fact, this rigidity is due to a general mobility of the thorax based on innumerable "micromovements." The articular components contained in the thorax are able to absorb considerable physical shock during sudden external impact or other trauma, thereby protecting the organs enclosed. As my colleague Pierre Mercier has noted, the general axis of the thorax (the resultant of the axes of individual thoracic structures) passes through the anterior heart and the ascending aorta. As movement near this axis is limited, the heart is not subject to any significant compression or stretching during thoracic movements.

Manual medicine tends to emphasize vertebral articulations at the expense of other thoracic articulations, even though the latter are more vulnerable to trauma. One of our aims in this book is to describe and analyze the entire thoracic osteoarticular system as a basis for teaching appropriate manipulation in this area. In *Visceral Manipulation* and *Visceral Manipulation II*, we discussed thoracoabdominal communications at length, stressing the diaphragmatic hiatus and the gastroesophageal junction. In this book, our interest lies more with the cervicothoracic junction and its complex myofascial layers.

Vascular problems of the thoracic inlet are quite common. Spinal manipulation in these cases can be useful but is usually insufficient. This is because the entire circulatory system in this area is dependent on the fasciae which surround the wide veins and lymphatic vessels and help keep them open. Thus, a restriction of the middle cervical aponeurosis can cause debilitating vertebrobasilar problems, which cannot be entirely resolved by osteoarticular treatments. Another common example is the sequelae of motor vehicle accidents, when the cervicopleural attachments are stretched, creating pleural restrictions. These pleural restrictions are what restrict cervical articular movements.

In such cases, it is better to manipulate the suspensory ligaments of the pleura rather than the cervical spine.

In preparing this book we made extensive use of dissections in order to avoid being restricted by purely theoretical concepts. The effects we observed of various types of trauma or respiratory conditions on the soft tissues of the thorax were impressive. However, dissections of non-living tissues can never be as instructive as daily clinical practice—we have always affirmed that the "hands take precedence." A suffering patient is not an equation to be solved with pen and paper. The techniques described in this book have been used repeatedly, and their effectiveness proven, in a clinical setting.

As in our previous books, we have availed ourselves of imaging technology. For example, in this book we utilize CT scans to prove that the thoracic inlet is naturally narrower during certain movements. Experiments utilizing Doppler devices, which we performed in 1985 with the help of Morzol Bernard, showed us the efficiency of certain techniques and also the extreme variability of effects due to vascular compression of this inlet. From one day to the next, and even from one hour to the next, depending on sleeping or working position, emotional state, hormonal conditions, etc., subclavian arterial flow can be more or less disturbed. Physicians often attribute related symptoms to depression because of the lack of easily reproducible objective signs. Observations we made at the Radiology Clinic of Grenoble utilizing the CT scanner and the expertise of Alain Dubreuil clearly show that very little is needed to produce functional restriction of blood vessels in the cervicothoracic area. We need to be particularly careful when drawing conclusions from Doppler exams involving these blood vessels. We have seen many times that even minor restrictions of the tissues, which might be harmless elsewhere, have significant effects in the cervicothoracic area, e.g., producing compression of vascular systems having large diameter and flow volume.

For all these reasons, we must emphasize the importance of knowing how to examine and treat the thorax and its contents.

Chapter One: *Overview*

Table of Contents

CHAPTER ONE

Overview

Thoracic Anatomy

Inspection of the thorax leaves us with several paradoxical impressions. It appears superficially rigid, although we know that it contains countless articulations, all of which move with each respiration. It hides and protects essential organs (particularly the heart and lungs), while allowing them to remain in perpetual mobility and carry out their various functions.

The thorax communicates with adjacent body cavities via two openings—the cervicothoracic junction for the skull and the diaphragmatic hiatus for the abdomen. Of course, these openings are weak points where differing pressures and mechanical tensions constantly affect the soft tissues which surround and pass through the openings. We have already discussed structure and function of the diaphragmatic hiatus and gastroesophageal junction in *Visceral Manipulation* and *Visceral Manipulation II,* and will assume the reader's familiarity with these topics.

We shall now highlight certain key points concerning the thorax which will be discussed in greater detail in later chapters.

HARD FRAME

The hard frame of the thorax consists of bony elements such as the sternum, ribs, and spinal column. This frame contains at least *150* articulations, which give it surprising flexibility. For example, a typical rib contains or participates in a total of six articulations. Most practitioners of manual medicine focus their attention on the articulations of the spinal column at the expense of those elsewhere in the thorax, even though the latter are more exposed to trauma. With each respiration, all of the thoracic articulations are involved. A single restriction can disturb this complex mechanism, sometimes without causing any initial symptoms, because there are so many possible compensations. Each day, from normal respiration alone, the thoracic articulations collectively undergo more than three million movements. In addition, the heart by itself undergoes over one hundred thousand daily movements.

SOFT FRAME

The soft frame of the thorax consists of fasciae, ligaments, and visceral organs. Each organ is surrounded by a fascial system which protects it while allowing sufficient mobility. The soft frame is supported by and suspended from the hard frame. Therefore, any restriction of the bones can affect the organs, and vice versa. For example, an intercostal restriction can fix part of the pleura because of the relationship between the internal intercostal muscles, subcostal muscles, and pleura. The soft frame is fairly heavy (the lungs weigh 1.3 kg); however, intrathoracic subatmospheric pressure enables the lungs to exert an effective traction of only a few hundred grams.

VISCERAL FRAME

The visceral frame of the thorax, consisting of the heart and lungs, is characterized by high mobility because both of these organs move constantly and with relatively large amplitudes. Any injury to its support or suspensory systems will eventually result in serious organic pathology. However, these organs can also develop intrinsic pathologies, which we will discuss later. We are uncertain about the significance of other thoracic organs (e.g., thymus) in visceral manipulation, and have not been able to prove the efficacy of our techniques aimed at these organs. Release of a costal or pleural restriction causes an immediate and easily-documented improvement of respiratory amplitude, but how can we demonstrate an effect on the thymus? Our dissections have shown us how vestigial this organ is in adults, and it is difficult for us to conceive of any effect based on "pumping the thymus."

Origins of Thoracic Restrictions

Thoracic restrictions generally result from mechanical, infectious, or tumoral problems, which can be very interdependent. Diagnosis is often difficult. Take the example of left thoracic pain, localized around the fourth rib. Is it a problem of the breast, heart, lung, or fourth rib? We are often confronted by this type of situation. In this section, we will discuss several categories of problems affecting the thorax.

OBSTETRIC

Sustained malpositioning of the fetus within the uterus may result in scoliosis deforming the thorax and causing problems of the thoracic inlet and hiatus. For example, children born in a breech position often suffer from congenital torticollis. This torticollis is more of a restriction of the cervicothoracic junction, which can be difficult to diagnose initially. The head is held in sidebending and rotation, always toward the same side. These children often have positive Adson-Wright tests. They may subsequently develop thoracic outlet syndrome with imbalance of the cervicopleural attachments, which can lead to cervical pain or "idiopathic" cervicobrachial neuralgia. We see many such cases. Usually, questioning reveals no history of specific trauma. In these cases any apparent effectiveness of cervical manipulation is deceptive; both the pain and the restrictions will quickly recur. Manipulation of the upper thorax will, however, quickly bring about long-lasting relief.

TRAUMATIC

Traumas which can affect thoracic function include falls on or blows to the shoulder, chest, and back. The neck is more mobile than the thorax, and restrictions are more common near the cervicothoracic junction than elsewhere in the cervical spine. Such restrictions are often very deeply located, near the first rib. Since lower cervical restrictions typically disturb the cervicopleural system and upper thoracic fascia, it is important to test the inside of the supraclavicular fossa, as will be explained below.

Motor vehicle accidents provoke multiple thoracic restrictions, particularly when the subject was wearing a seat-belt. Although it undeniably saves lives in many cases, the seat-belt can also cause upper thoracic restrictions which are very complex and difficult to treat. The thorax is highly deformable and because of its multiple articulations has a remarkable ability to compensate for trauma, even a major auto crash. Nonetheless, the restrictions gradually make themselves known, sometimes several years after the accident, often to the great surprise of the patient himself.

VISCERAL

All visceral pathologies affect the thorax, sometimes in unexpected and interesting ways. We often treat young athletes who come because of cervicoscapular pain after running several kilometers. Mobility tests are normal except for tense, fixed cervicopleural ligaments. Questioning and listening tests reveal old lesions from pulmonary tuberculosis. Analysis of such cases has shown us that running increases myofascial tensions, as well as respiratory rhythm and amplitude. The pleura therefore pulls more on its attachments. Because tubercular lesions are found near the apex of the lungs, the superior attachment system has already suffered, and lost its elasticity and distensibility. This example, like many others, shows that the dividing line between visceral and mechanical problems is tenuous at best.

SURGICAL

After thoracic surgery there is obviously an imbalance of thoracic mobility due to the concentration and focusing of forces on a particular zone of the fascial system. However, even abdominopelvic and other types of surgery have destabilizing effects on the thorax. We have seen many patients having one operation after another, e.g., initially for the bladder, one year later for an inguinal hernia, and two years later for a hiatal hernia. As osteopaths, we see this as due to a loss of proper reciprocal tension in the body due to disruption caused by the surgery. Even for gastroesophageal reflux, a common cause of respiratory problems, one must treat all surgical scars within the body, because any one can destabilize the attachments of the cardia.

INFECTIOUS

The lungs are a favorite target of infectious organisms which attack the human body. Our dissections have shown us how often these attacks take place. Each infection leaves scar tissue, which disturbs pleuropulmonary mobility in general. It has been suggested (though without definitive proof) that vaccinations, in spite of their protective function, can cause parenchymatous lesions and lead to predisposition of certain areas to infection. It is true that we have seen some young patients who developed pleuropulmonary restrictions after vaccination. These restrictions were detected using listening techniques, and were not present before the vaccination. Such observations, of course, do not allow us to confirm or deny the hypothesis mentioned above. Individuals react differently to vaccinations, and restrictions can arise for many reasons.

Pollution must be mentioned as a possible cause of thoracic restrictions, since it initially attacks the respiratory system. It is certainly a common cause of pulmonary lesions, and predisposes the respiratory system to a variety of diseases.

TUMORS

As you know, the lungs and thorax are subject to numerous types of tumors, both primary and secondary, which are spread via the lymphatic system or bloodstream. Lung and breast cancers are the types of cancer most likely to cause death in women, and lung cancer is also a leading source of mortality in men. (Cancer symptoms and diagnosis will be discussed in greater detail in Chapter 4.) Sooner or later in your practice, you will find yourself dealing with a patient who has a tumor. In the initial stages, tumors often present with symptoms that are unremarkable and can easily be confused with those of less serious diseases.

Vascular Effects of Thoracic Inlet Restrictions

Most thoracic restrictions have an effect on the vascular system of the inlet. The thoracic inlet is naturally narrow and all the components within it are compressed. A minor restriction whose counterpart in the abdominal cavity would be harmless becomes significant here. The subclavian artery is an important element in this area, but we must not neglect the veins and lymphatic vessels. Although physical examinations typically emphasize the arterial system, our own studies (confirmed by CT scanning) show that it is the venous system which initially suffers from compression in the inlet. The symptoms are less obvious but just as debilitating as those of arterial compression. In Chapter 2 we shall discuss the role of fasciae (particularly the middle cervical aponeurosis) in venous circulation of the inlet. This aponeurosis is crucial to our ability to obtain effective results in treatment of the vascular system in this area.

Chapter Two: Applied Anatomy

Table of Contents

Applied Anatomy

As in our previous books, our goal here is not to fill up several pages with detailed, textbook-style information. We assume that you already know your anatomy, and will concern ourselves only with emphasizing important points and various peculiarities which we consider indispensable to the understanding of mobility tests and treatment. For convenience, we shall examine the systems in sequence: osteoarticular, fascial, muscular, visceral, and neurovascular. You should keep in mind, of course, that functions of these systems are integrated and interdependent.

In anatomical discussion, we tend to rely on authors from the nineteenth century and earlier because they were very close to actual anatomy and just reported and drew what they saw. Many modern authors oversimplify (and sometimes actually change) anatomy in order to make drawings which they consider more aesthetically pleasing. Of course, we also base our discussions on the dissections which we have performed ourselves.

Osteoarticular System

This system of bones and cartilage encloses and protects the visceral and neurovascular systems. The osteoarticular system is closely related to the organs. For example, a restriction of the sternoclavicular joint may affect the heart, lungs, or vascular system.

STERNOCLAVICULAR JOINT

This consists of a fibrocartilaginous articular meniscus. The sternal facet faces superolaterally and slightly posteriorly, while the clavicular facet is directed inferomedially and slightly anteriorly. The clavicles reinforce the upper part of the sternum and prevent it from becoming concave inward.

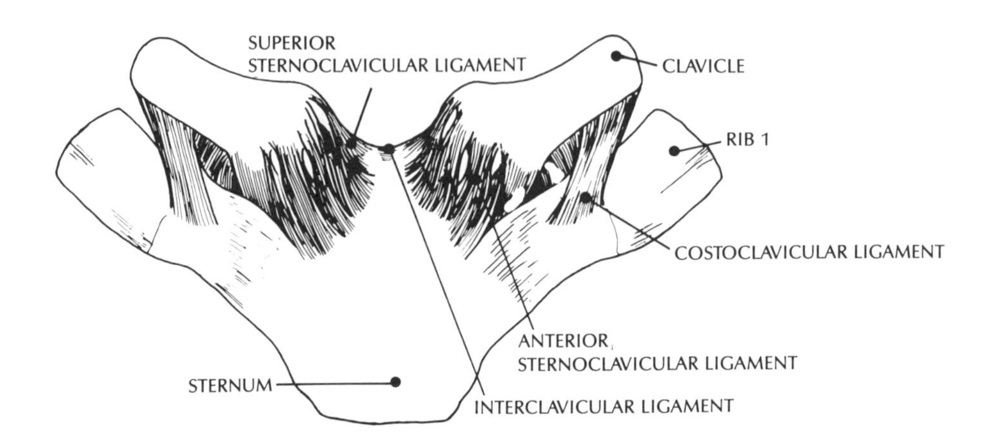

Illustration 2-1
Sternoclavicular Joint (after Testut & Jacob)

The sternoclavicular joint is supported by four ligaments (Illustration 2-1):

- An anterior sternoclavicular ligament, the middle fasciculi being the firmest.
- A posterior sternoclavicular ligament, the fibers running inferomedially. This ligament is related to the sternohyoid and sternothyroid muscles.
- An interclavicular ligament, running transversely under the clavicles. It is actually the joining of the two superior clavicular ligaments. It unites the superior and posterior parts of the medial clavicular extremities by partly filling the concavity of the sternal notch. Its posterior part corresponds to the sternothyroid muscle. This ligament is stretched when the shoulder is lowered, a characteristic which we use in both testing and treatment of the sternoclavicular joint. The presence of this ligament requires that whenever there is a restriction of one side of the articulation, we treat both sides.
- A costoclavicular ligament running inferomedially from the clavicle to the first costal cartilage. It is divided into two layers, anterior and posterior, and there may be a serous bursa between the two. The presence of this ligament in theory renders the sternoclavicular and first sternocostal joints interdependent. However, certain traumas, e.g., a fall onto the shoulders or compression due to a seat-belt, can create clavicular restrictions without costal restrictions, or vice versa.

We believe that the sternoclavicular joint is one of the important crossroads of the body. Superiorly it is related to the hyoid via the middle cervical aponeurosis. This in turn gives it a strong connection to the cranium. Inferiorly it is related to the pleura. We will see later the importance these relationships have in the pathogenesis and treatment of disease.

ACROMIOCLAVICULAR JOINT

In about 33% of the population, this joint contains an intra-articular meniscus.

The clavicular facet faces inferolaterally, the acromial facet superomedially. The capsule is relatively loose, although the joint is supported by various ligaments as described below.

Acromioclavicular Ligaments

These run transversely and parallel to the plane of the clavicle, and tend to reinforce this bone. The posterior fibers are stronger and divided into superior and inferior portions. The inferior portion shares fibers with the conoid ligament (see below).

Coracoclavicular Ligaments

These are frequently overlooked, though significant, structures, and are involved in various restrictions of the thorax. It is important to clearly visualize their orientation (Illustrations 2-2 and 2-3).

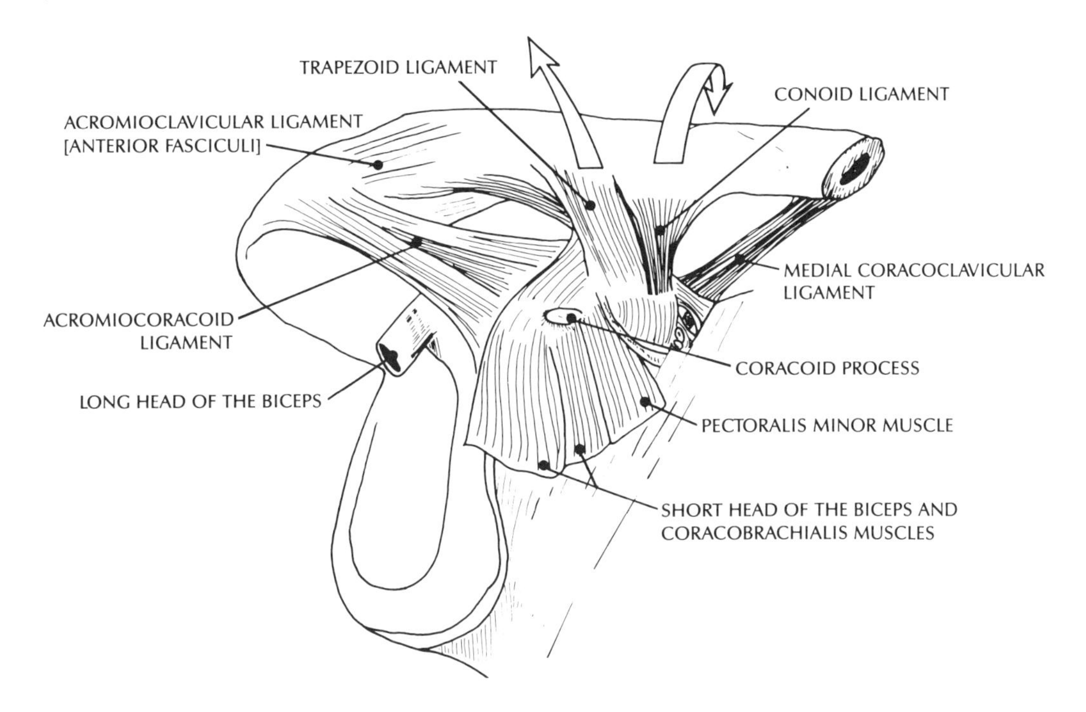

Illustration 2-2
Orientation of the Coracoclavicular Ligaments: Anterior View (after Testut & Jacob)

The *trapezoid ligament* is a fibrous blade of 3-6mm in thickness that is oriented primarily in the sagittal plane as it runs superolaterally from the posteromedial part of the coracoid process of the scapula to the anterior aspect of the clavicle. The *conoid ligament* is oriented on a frontal plane and runs posterosuperiorly and medially. These two ligaments join together and, with the inferior surface of the clavicle, form a kind of pocket filled with soft tissue. The lateral edge of the subclavius muscle is contiguous with this pocket and exchanges fibers with these ligaments.

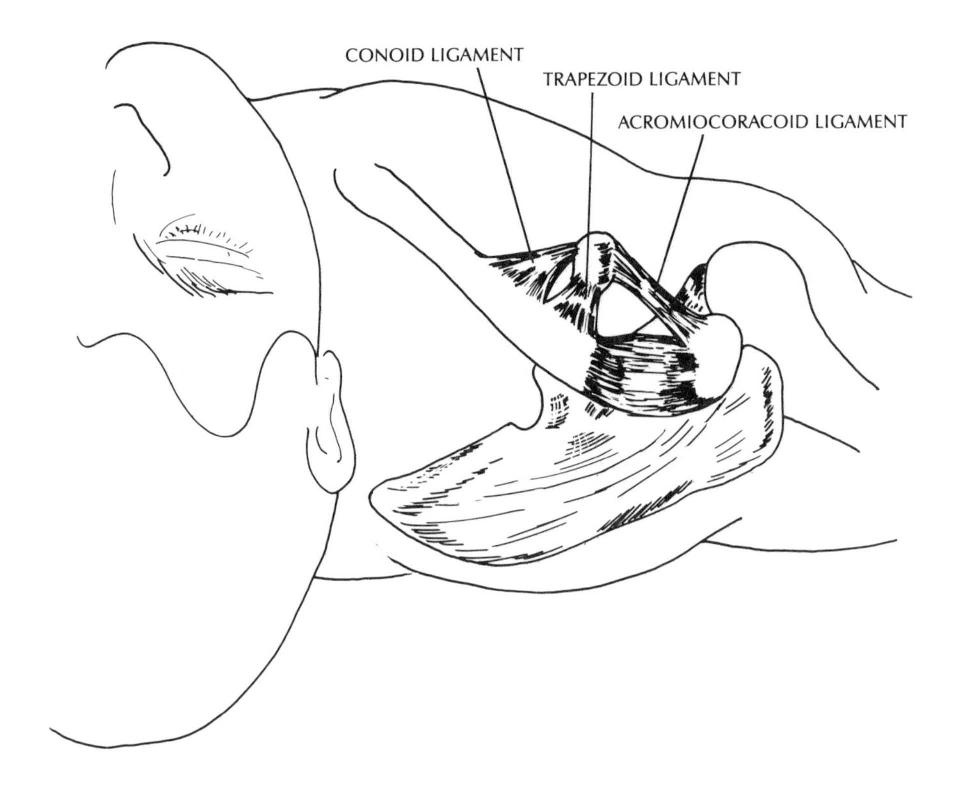

Illustration 2-3
Orientation of the Coracoclavicular Ligaments: Superior View

The *medial coracoclavicular ligament* is a thin, fibrous bundle running from the superior side of the coracoid process of the scapula along the anterior groove of the subclavius muscle, where it unites with the muscle's aponeurosis. For this reason, treatment of this aponeurosis should include stretching the coracoclavicular ligaments.

Acromiocoracoid Ligament

This runs from the inferior part of the summit of the acromion process to the edge of the coracoid process of the scapula. It is shaped like a triangle with anterior, middle and posterior fasciculi, and runs posterosuperiorly and laterally. There is a serous bursa between this ligament and the humeral capsule. Some authors do not consider this structure a true ligament because, together with the acromion and coracoid processes, it forms an osteofibrous dome which partially surrounds the scapulohumeral articulation. However, our observations indicate that it is often fixed in cases of direct or indirect trauma to the shoulder, and functions as a ligament.

INTRASTERNAL JOINTS

The sternum is a very important bone that is neglected by most practitioners of manipulation. For us perhaps its most important function is the distribution throughout the chest of the forces of chest trauma. Originally, the sternum is composed of many bones which become fused into three by adulthood: the manubrium, body, and xiphoid process. These three are connected by two rudimentary joints: the sternomanubrial and sternoxiphoid.

The *sternomanubrial joint* contains an interosseous ligament which disappears only in very old age. This is found at the level of the second sternocostal articulation, near the sternal angle, and can be fixed as a result of direct trauma to the chest, e.g., impact with the dashboard or seat-belt during a car crash. These restrictions almost always involve associated sternochondral or superior costochondral problems. The fibrocartilage of the sternomanubrial joint can be compared to the intervertebral discs. They are continuous externally with the interosseous ligament and second sternochondral joint. Sometimes there is a real articular fissure, surrounded by a capsule.

The *sternoxiphoid joint* is more rudimentary, since the xiphoid process is reduced in humans. Restrictions here are rare, but may cause gastroesophageal or other digestive problems when they do occur.

STERNOCHONDRAL AND COSTOCHONDRAL JOINTS

The sternum articulates directly with the costal cartilages of ribs 1-7 (but not ribs 8-12). These *sternochondral joints* can be considered as gliding joints. They consist of a capsule, a fibrous cuff derived from the costal perichondrium, an anteriorly radiating ligament, and an interosseous ligament. The superior and inferior fibers of these ligaments intersect with those of the neighboring ligaments; the middle fibers merge with those of the opposite side (Illustration 2-4). Thus, restriction of a sternochondral joint almost always affects the joint opposite as well as those above and below. The tracts

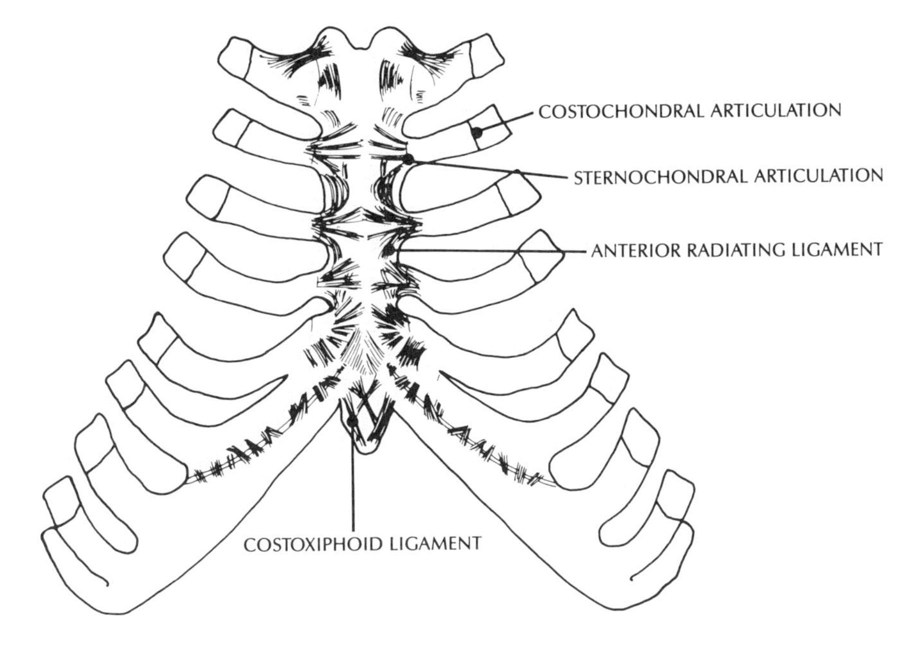

Illustration 2-4
Sternochondral and Costochondral Joints (after Charpy)

of the anterior radiating ligament mix with the tendinous origin of the pectoralis major muscle, which explains the frequent costal restrictions of gymnasts and physical laborers. There are several bunches of fibers on the posterior side of these joints. The seventh costochondral is reinforced by the costoxiphoid ligaments. The interosseous ligament stretches from the costal crest to the cartilage of each rib. When people become old, the sternal periosteum, which joins the perichondrium of the costal cartilages, becomes ossified.

Costochondral joints are, in our view, synarthroses which join the ribs to the costal cartilages. These joints, because of their elasticity, play an important role in large-scale movements of the thorax. We sometimes find cartilaginous fixations here which cannot be neglected because of the mechanical disturbances which they cause, even in the elderly. Many anatomists dismiss the idea of costochondral articular problems. However, we place greater faith in conclusions based on examination of live patients than in those based on dissections. Our clinical experience continually shows us problems related to these joints, or at least to their ligaments.

Muscular System

We are concerned here mainly with smaller thoracic muscles which we use for treatment of intrathoracic and extrathoracic problems. The large muscles are of relatively little interest to us. Problems affecting them are almost always secondary, i.e., due to an "overflow" or cascade of decompensations arising from dysfunctions elsewhere in the body. Large muscles are very rarely responsible for primary restrictions, and treating them gives a transient response at best. For example, a restriction of the trapezius muscle will have little general effect—apart from rare cases of a myofibril tear of traumatic origin. Problems with this muscle are typically a reflection of psychological tensions. Stretching the trapezius muscle can lead to a satisfactory relaxation, but it does not last long.

In addition, it is our experience that small muscles retain the "memory" of trauma much longer than large muscles and therefore have a greater overall effect on the body. When large muscles are affected by trauma, they show a relatively strong but brief reaction. Sometimes there is actual scarring, but this does not have much effect on the body. For these reasons, we prefer to work on restrictions of small muscles, e.g., subclavius, which are more likely to be both pathogenic and primary.

SUBCLAVIUS

Although this muscle is overlooked by many practitioners, the consequences of contracture or fibrosis here are considerable. The thoracic inlet is naturally very narrow. Disturbance of the surrounding muscular system (which includes the subclavius) may further narrow this opening and interfere with normal blood flow.

The subclavius is a roughly cylindrical muscle located underneath the clavicle, originating from the cartilage of rib 1 and from the most medial part of the bone (Illustration 2-5). The muscular fibers go superolaterally and posteriorly, inserting on the middle part of the inferior clavicle. The orientation is about the same as that of the costoclavicular ligament. The lateral fibers insert via a strong tendon between the conoid and trapezoid ligaments. It is therefore impossible to manipulate the subclavius muscle without also manipulating these two ligaments. In some people, the muscle is attached to the coracoid process instead of the clavicle.

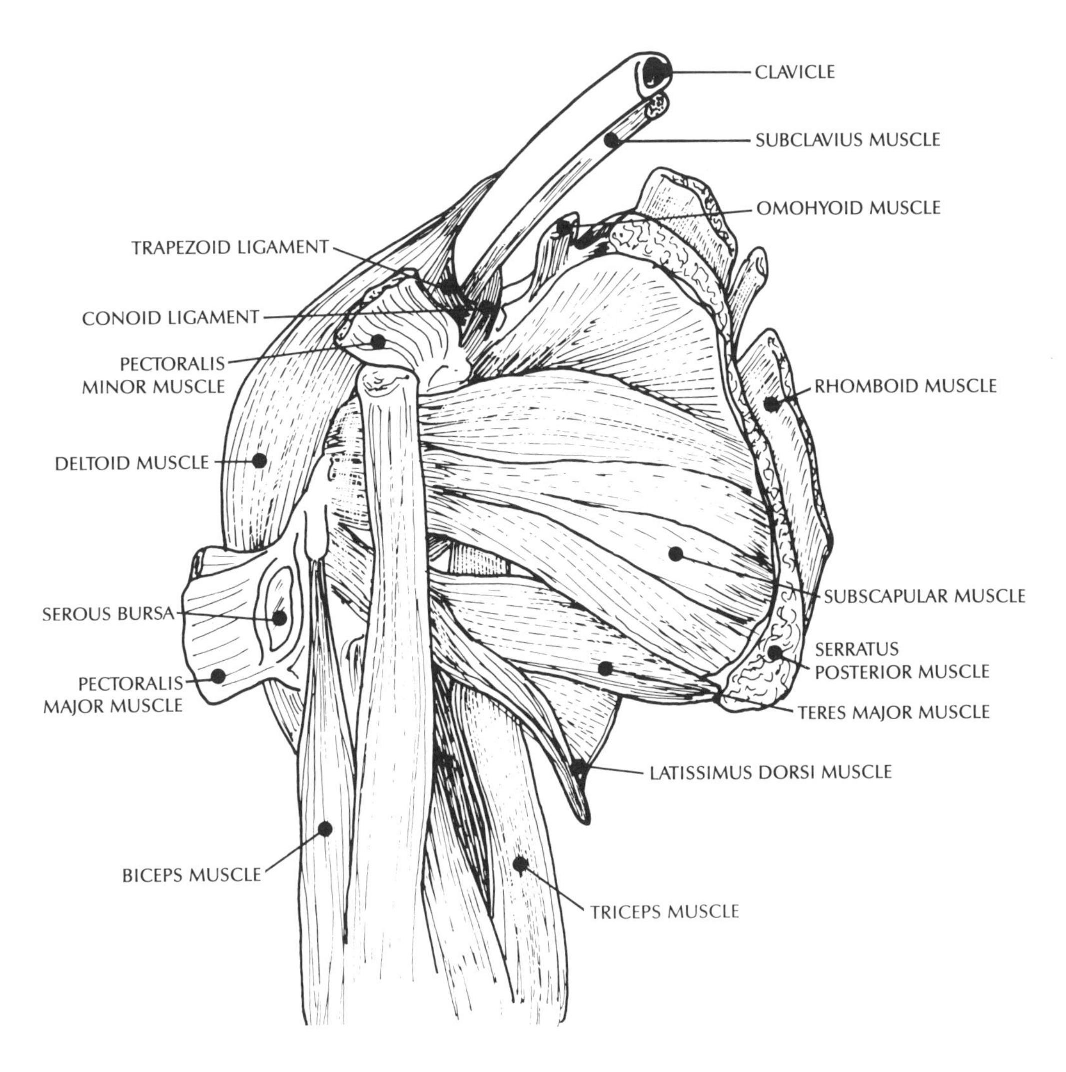

Illustration 2-5
Subclavious Muscle and Its Relationship to the Conoid and Trapezoid Ligaments (after Clemente)

The subclavius lowers the clavicle and shoulder or, if the shoulder is fixed, elevates rib 1 during inhalation. It also functions as a ligament of the sternoclavicular joint. The muscle is innervated by cervical nerves 5 and 6 via the brachial plexus. Fibers of these nerves anastomose with the phrenic nerve, which explains why irritations of the phrenic nerve often affect the subclavius. Such irritations can be of visceral (lungs, liver, bladder) or peritoneal origin, since the peritoneum is partially innervated by the superior part of the phrenic nerve.

Anteriorly, the subclavius is covered by the clavipectoral fascia and pectoralis major muscle. Posteriorly, it is separated from rib 1 by the subclavian vessels and brachial plexus. It is near the origin of the sternothyroid muscle, which runs along the posterior clavicle.

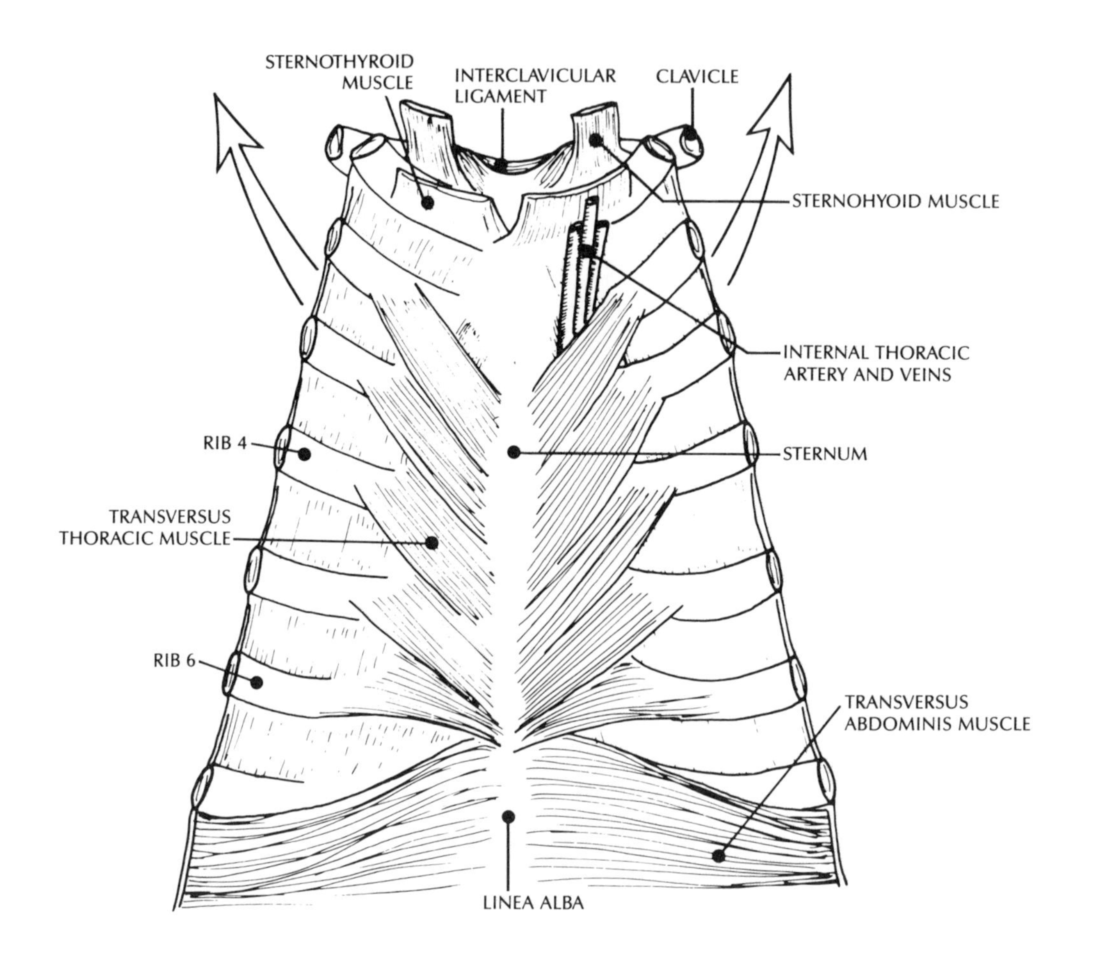

Illustration 2-6
Transversus Thoracic Muscle (after Charpy & Nicolas)

TRANSVERSUS THORACIS

This thin, fan-shaped muscle has a large fascial component. It originates with a short aponeurosis from the lower third of the posterior sternal body, xiphoid process, and costochondral joints of ribs 5-7 (sometimes rib 4). The fibers run superolaterally to insert on the inferior and internal surfaces of the costal cartilages of ribs 3-6 (sometimes rib 2) (Illustration 2-6). The inferior transverse digitations, which arise from rib 6, are continuous with the superior tract of the transversus abdominis muscle.

Posteriorly, the transversus thoracis relates and adheres to the parietal layer of the anterior pleural pouch. Some consider it mainly an exhalatory muscle, but we have noticed that it can become fixed during pleuropulmonary problems, in turn affecting the sternochondral and costochondral joints. As such it may be considered a tensor of the pleura. Restrictions of this muscle can be the cause of dull intrathoracic pain not accountable to other factors. Due to its connection with the transversus abdominis, it can also be affected by certain peritoneal irritations.

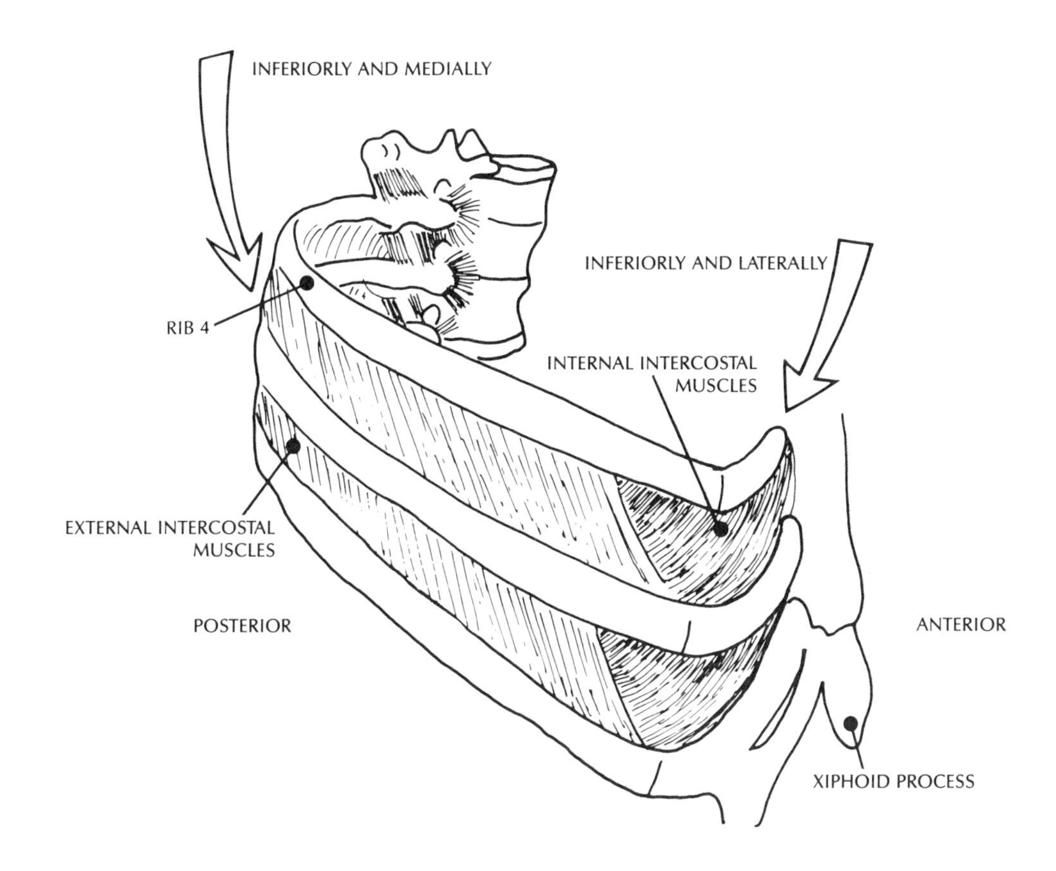

Illustration 2-7
Intercostal Muscles

INTERCOSTALS AND SUBCOSTALS

There are eleven pairs of external and internal intercostal muscles (Illustration 2-7). The *external intercostals* run from the costotransverse joints posteriorly to the level of the costochondral joints anteriorly, where their fleshy fibers become aponeurotic. They have an anteroinferior orientation. The *internal intercostals* run from the sternum (or the anterior extremities of costochondrals 8-10) to end near the posterior angles of the ribs. They have a close relationship with the endothoracic aponeurosis and pleura, and are oriented posteroinferiorly. The intercostal muscles are continuous with the external and internal oblique muscles of the abdomen.

The *subcostal* muscles are found between the costal pleura and the internal intercostals, and have a large fascial component. Generally found only on the middle and lower ribs, they originate from the internal surface of one rib to insert on the internal surface of the second or third rib down. Together with the transversus thoracis, they merge inferiorly with the transversus abdominis muscle. Like the internal intercostals, their orientation is posteroinferior.

The intercostals seem to serve a modulatory role during major respiratory movements. They function as a kind of "thoracic drum," damping large pressure variations, notably during coughing or sneezing. They are almost always sclerosed in pleural disorders, as we have demonstrated during dissection. The subcostal muscles are thought by some researchers to play a role in pleural tension.

LEVATORES COSTARUM

These muscles have a short, flat, triangular shape. They run from the transverse processes of C7 and T1-11 to the twelve ribs, and are divided into two groups. The *short levatores costarum* muscles run from the tip of the transverse process to the rib which is directly underneath (Illustration 2-8). The first goes from C7 to rib 1, and the last from T11 to rib 12. The *long levatores costarum* muscles are more lateral and located mostly in the inferior intercostal spaces. They start from the transverse process, jump one or two intercostal spaces, and insert on the posterior angle of the rib. There are generally four—the first going from the transverse process of T7 to rib 9, and the last from T10 to rib 12.

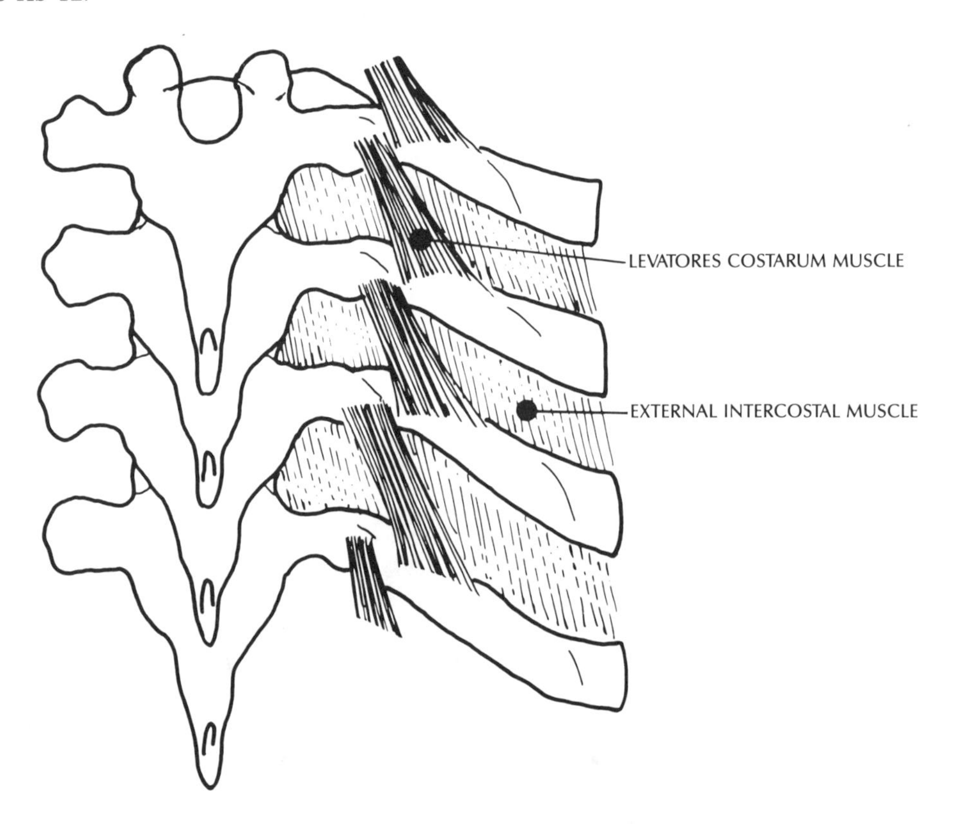

Illustration 2-8
Levatores Costarum Muscles (after Charpy & Nicolas)

We mention these muscles because we often find that they are fixed with pleuropulmonary problems. In these cases, mobility tests of the spinal column are usually negative. The ribs are fixed at the level of the posterior angles rather than the costovertebral joints, and it is therefore difficult to push the costal angle anterolaterally.

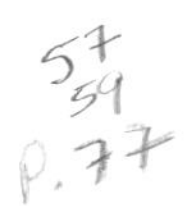

DIAPHRAGM

We shall mention this principal inhalatory muscle only briefly. One can certainly not deny its important role, but we are not convinced that restrictions of the diaphragm, either one-sided or total, are pathogenic. Like all the large muscles, the diaphragm is one of the structures that handles "overflows" of tension. It may become fixed by various imbalances of either psychological or metabolic origins. Symptoms, which result from limitations of the track of the hemidiaphragm or whole diaphragm, include a heavy feeling in the area between the thorax and abdomen, shallow breathing, and difficulty with inhalation. The patient should be advised to begin relaxation or stretching techniques. Some helpful stretches include sidebending and rotating the last six ribs, along with forward/backward bending and sidebending of T12, L1, and L2.

In osteopathy, restrictions of the hemidiaphragm are almost always dependent upon a malfunction of the ipsilateral viscera, or upon a vertebral or costal restriction. Hypomobility of the whole diaphragm is, however, more likely to be related to a psychological problem or general weakness. When T12-L2 are fixed, vertebral manipulations may have a beneficial effect on the diaphragm.

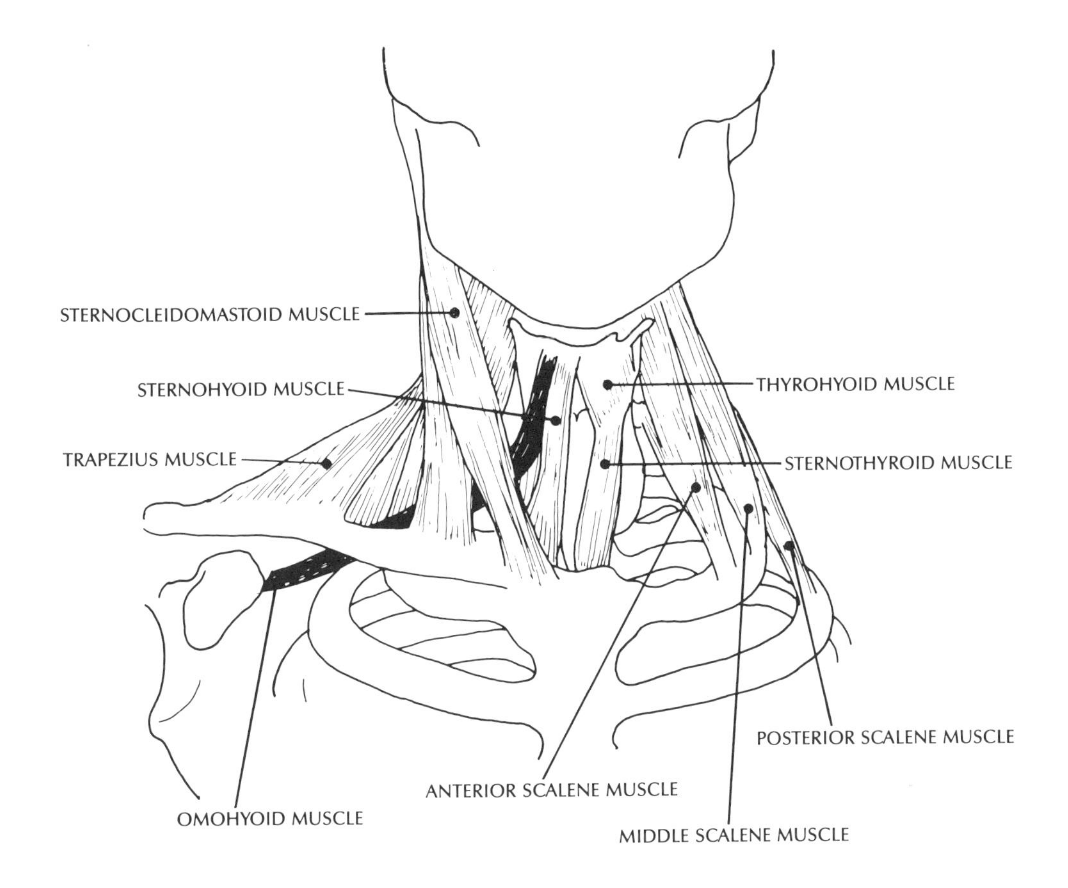

Illustration 2-9
Subhyoid Muscles (after Charpy & Nicolas)

INFRAHYOIDS

These have a fascial as well as a muscular role, i.e., serving to reinforce the action of the middle cervical aponeurosis. There are four infrahyoid muscles, divided into superficial and deep groups. The superficial group includes the sternohyoid and omohyoid, often considered as essentially the same muscle. The middle part of this muscle becomes progressively more fibrous until it is called the middle cervical aponeurosis. The deep group comprises the sternothyroid and thyrohyoid (Illustration 2-9).

The *sternohyoid* arises from the posterior side of the medial end of the clavicle, and from the costoclavicular ligament and sternum. It runs superomedially to insert on the inferior edge of the hyoid bone. The *omohyoid* originates from the superior scapula just inside the coracoid notch, and runs superomedially to the inferior hyoid. It is sheathed by the middle cervical aponeurosis with which it exchanges fibers. The *sternothyroid* comes from the posterior sides of the sternum and first costal cartilage, and from several fibers of the second costal cartilage. It runs superolaterally to insert on the two tubercles on the lateral thyroid cartilage, and exchanges a few fibers with the sternohyoid muscle. The *thyrohyoid* is an extension of the sternothyroid, running from the thyroid cartilage to the hyoid bone.

Contraction of these muscles lowers the hyoid bone. More importantly, they can fix the hyoid, thereby assisting in depression of the mandible. They also have a fascial role in tensing the middle cervical aponeurosis, which allows the damping of large changes in pressure levels which could have an effect on the cervicothoracic venous system.

SCALENES

These muscles are well known, and we will only remind you of their insertions in order to later clarify certain particularities (Illustration 2-10).

The *anterior scalene* runs from the anterior tubercles of the transverse processes of C3-6, to the scalene tubercle on the superior edge of rib 1, 2-3cm from its medial extremity. The *middle scalene* runs from the transverse processes of C2-8 to the superolateral surface of rib 1. The *posterior scalene* runs from the transverse processes of C4-6 to the superior edge of rib 2.

The sheath of the anterior scalene unites with that of the subclavius muscle to surround the subclavian vein. Therefore, every treatment of the subclavius should be accompanied by stretching of the anterior scalene.

Fascial System

The thoracic fascial system is quite important in osteopathy and we shall discuss it in some detail. In addition to its more obvious roles, it also functions as a tensor of the pleura and as a venolymphatic activator during respiration.

The aponeuroses are of varying degrees of importance and we will discuss them on the basis of their osteopathic relevance. We have never been able to demonstrate a noteworthy effect from a restriction of the superficial fascia. Those of you who have had the opportunity to observe it during dissection know that it is as thin as a sheet of cellophane, and probably too thin to have much widespread effect. Certain aponeuroses (the middle cervical, clavipectoral, and pleura) deserve greater attention because their restrictions can cause significant disturbances elsewhere.

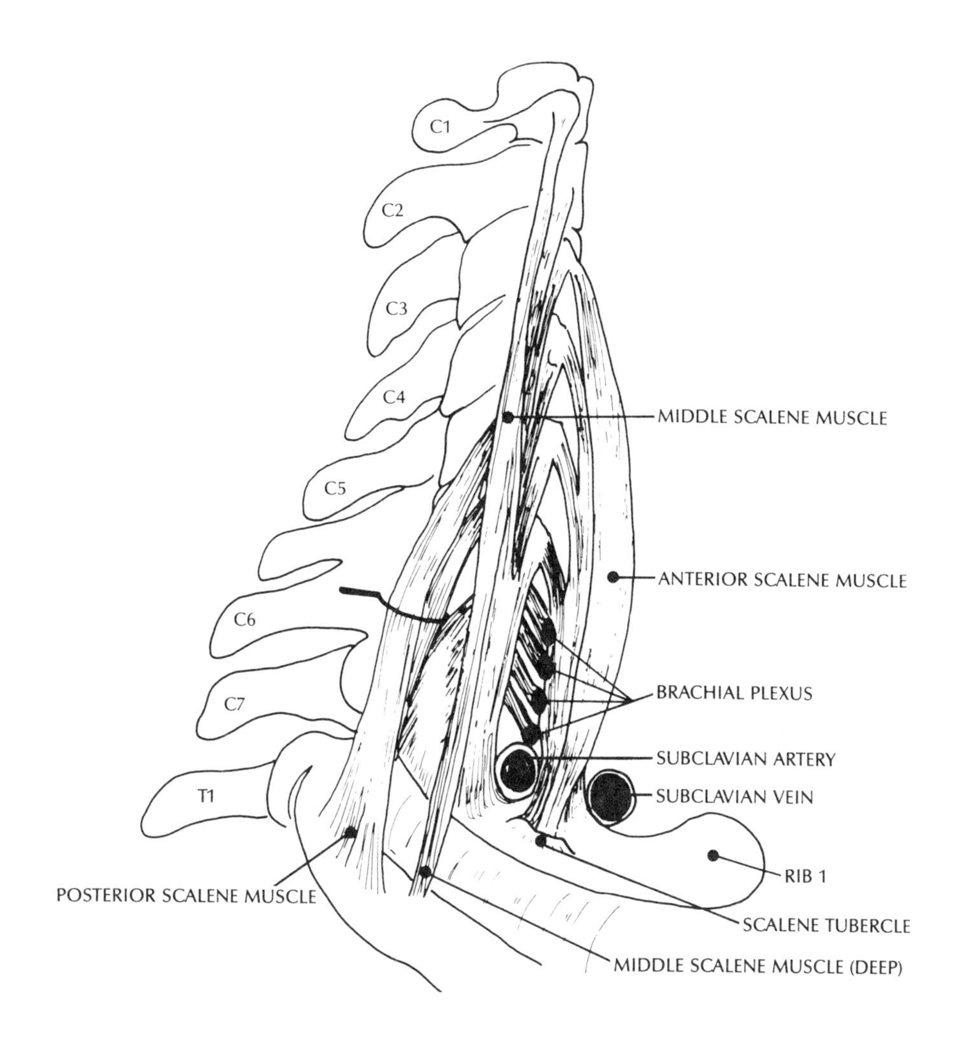

Illustration 2-10
Scalene Muscles (after Charpy & Nicolas)

SUPERFICIAL CERVICAL FASCIA AND PLATYSMA MUSCLE

Clinical experience has shown us few points of osteopathic interest regarding the *superficial cervical fascia.* Like all superficial fasciae, is it essentially a layer of disorganized loose connective tissue. It is superficial, thin, and has significant attachments only on the greater horn, inferior edge of the body, and process of the hyoid bone.

The *platysma muscle* arises from the fascia covering the upper parts of the pectoralis major and deltoid muscles. It crosses the clavicle and sternocleidomastoid, running superomedially along the side of the neck. Anteriorly, the fibers of one side interlace with those of the other along the midline. The more anterior fibers attach to the underside of the mandible; those farther posterior are attached to the skin and subcutaneous tissue of the lower part of the face. This muscle of facial expression also functions as an active aponeurosis which, through its variations of tonicity, attenuates the effects of atmospheric pressure on the external jugular vein and the veins entering the supraclavicular fossa. Its contraction enlarges the neck and dilates the vessels. It is less important than the middle cervical aponeurosis. The platysma muscle and superficial cervical fascia are closely associated.

MIDDLE CERVICAL APONEUROSIS

This aponeurosis also functions as the fascia of the infrahyoid muscles and as a part of the pretracheal fascia. Our experience shows that this is an essential element of the cervicothoracic junction. When it is restricted, there are adverse effects on the circulatory system. This aponeurosis runs from one omohyoid muscle to another. Its inferior insertion is on the upper border of the scapula near the scapular notch (the origin of the omohyoid muscle), posterior edge of the clavicle, scalene tubercle and cartilage of rib 1, medial extremity of the clavicle, and posterior sternum. At the top it inserts onto the hyoid bone (Illustrations 2-11 and 2-12).

One could say that it is attached to all the bony or fibrous surfaces of the thoracic inlet. We should emphasize its continuity with the aponeurosis of the subclavius muscle.

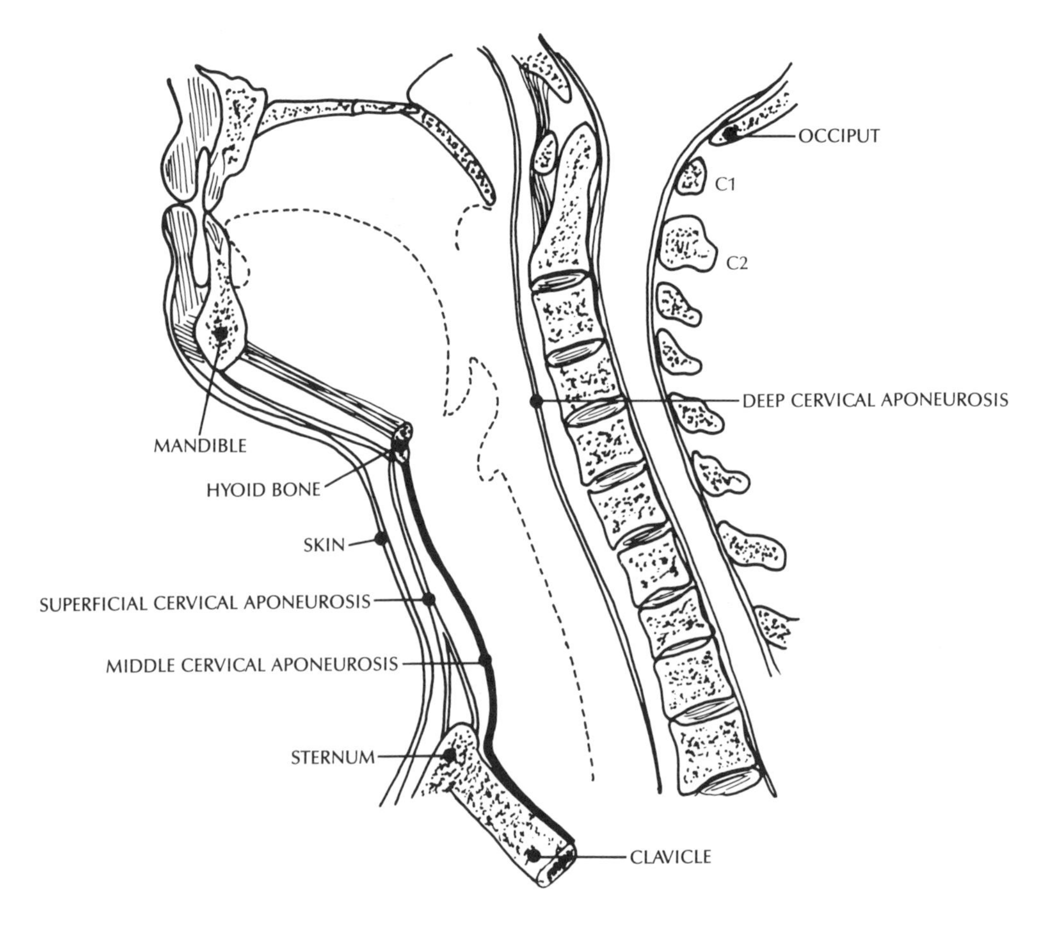

Illustration 2-11
Middle Cervical Aponeurosis: Sagittal Plane (after Testut & Jacob)

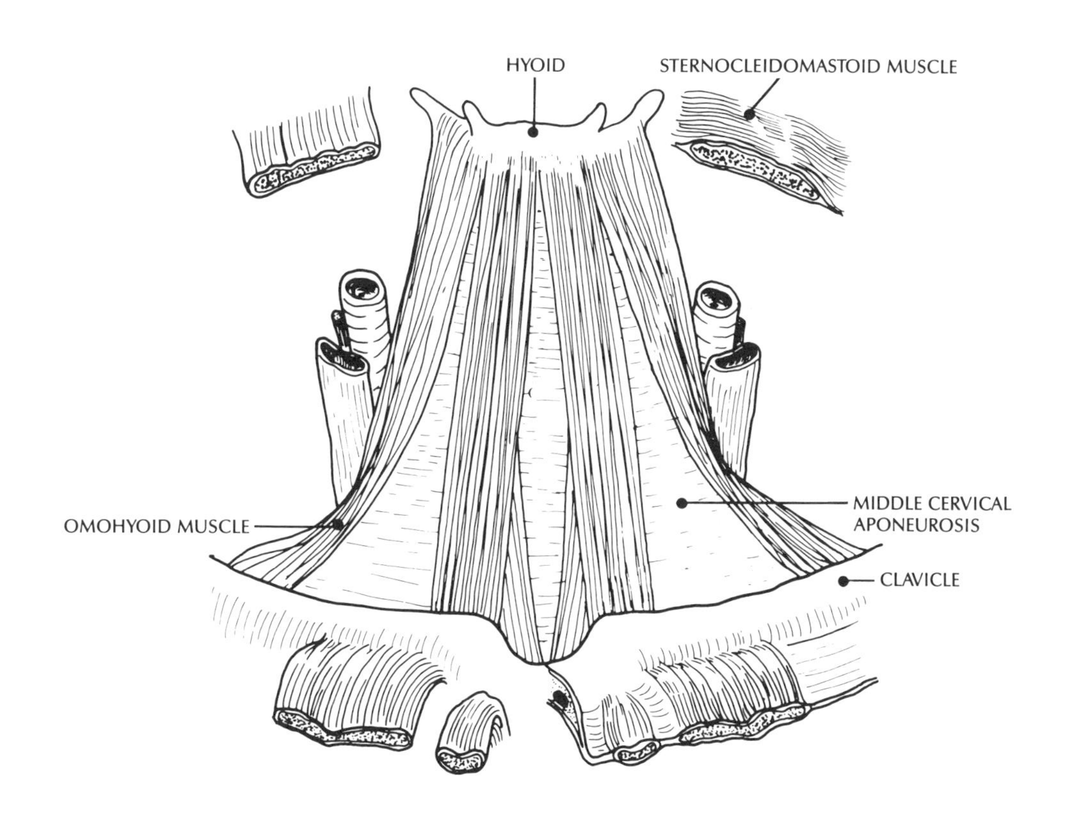

Illustration 2-12
Middle Cervical Aponeurosis: Frontal Plane (after Testut & Jacob)

It attaches above the sternohyoid muscles, and laterally to the anterior edge of the sternocleidomastoid muscle. This aponeurosis may contain muscular fibers, usually between the clavicle and omohyoid muscles. Its attachment at the scalene tubercle means that it not only exchanges fibers with the pleura and subclavius muscle, but also with the anterior scalene muscle.

Embryologically, it appears in the sixth fetal month. It seems to be the vestigial remnant of a muscle which connects the clavicle to the hyoid in other eutherian mammals.

In terms of function, the middle cervical aponeurosis does not seem to play a suspensory role for the pericardium and pleura. The superior sternopericardial ligament, discussed later, is attached to the posterior manubrium on the same line as the insertion of this aponeurosis. When the ligament is stretched, the pericardium is not lifted, but with adhesion and fibrosis the middle cervical aponeurosis may partially fix the pericardium.

We believe that this aponeurosis has two essential functions: muscular and circulatory.

Muscular: It supports the infrahyoid muscles in an optimal orientation. These long, thin muscles need such support to function properly.

Circulatory: The veins at the base of the neck cross through the middle cervical aponeurosis via fibrous canals. The aponeurosis surrounds all the large veins, i.e., brachiocephalic, thyroid, and subclavian. As the aponeurosis is fixed to bones (hyoid, clavicle, sternum) in several directions, it maintains the patency of the canals and consequently the veins, which are attached via fascial fibers. The middle cervical aponeurosis thus has the role of a lateral venal tensor. This opening of the veins accentuates the "inhalatory emptying" that promotes thoracic/cervical/cerebral venous circulation; i.e., the diameter of the veins increases with each inhalation because the first rib, sternum, and clavicle move away from each other. The aponeurosis is stretched mostly laterally and anteriorly, which tends to draw blood to the area, and its rigidity helps neutralize external pressure. When the aponeurosis is restricted the fixed points change. This can lead to a relative closure of some veins.

The inhalatory elevation of the upper thorax, superiorly and anteriorly, stretches not only the middle cervical aponeurosis, but also all the thoracic vascular sheaths. Tension of the aponeurosis can be accentuated by backward bending the neck. The aponeurosis is often affected by whiplash accidents, and we shall explain how to free it in order to reinstate good cervicothoracic and posterior cerebral venous circulation.

The vertebral vein is continuously open as it travels through the transverse foramina of the cervical vertebrae. It transmits the inhalatory "summons" to the diploe of the skull. A cervical restriction may interfere with opening of the vertebral vein and disturb its circulation.

DEEP CERVICAL APONEUROSIS

This aponeurosis, also known as the prevertebral fascia, represents the cervical continuation of the endothoracic fascia, transversalis, and pelvic fasciae. The deepest part goes from the occiput to T3, stretching from the anterior common vertebral ligament to the anterior tubercles of the transverse processes, and sometimes exchanges fibers with the dura mater.

This aponeurosis covers the posterior neck muscles which are organized in two groups on either side of the spinal column. The more medial group consists of the longus capitis and longus colli muscles, while the lateral group consists of the scalenes. The scalene sheath fixes itself to the anterior and posterior tubercles of the transverse process. Cervical nerves and numerous veins penetrate it as it runs to insert on rib 1. An aponeurotic expansion goes from the medial edge of the anterior scalene sheath to the anterior edge of the pleural dome. This expansion is part of the suspensory apparatus of the pleura and is sometimes called the scalenopleural ligament.

The inferior insertion of the anterior scalene muscle on the scalene tubercle is of great interest to us for two reasons: (1) some fibers of the sheath reinforce the aponeurosis of the subclavius muscle; (2) other fibers mix with the suspensory ligaments of the pleura. In osteopathy, these are both important structures.

SUBCLAVIAN APONEUROSIS

This solid aponeurosis attaches to the anterior clavicle and surrounds the subclavius muscle as it runs to the posterior clavicle. It constitutes the anterior, inferior, and posterior walls of the osteofibrous sheath of the subclavius muscle, the superior part being formed by the clavicle (Illustration 2-13).

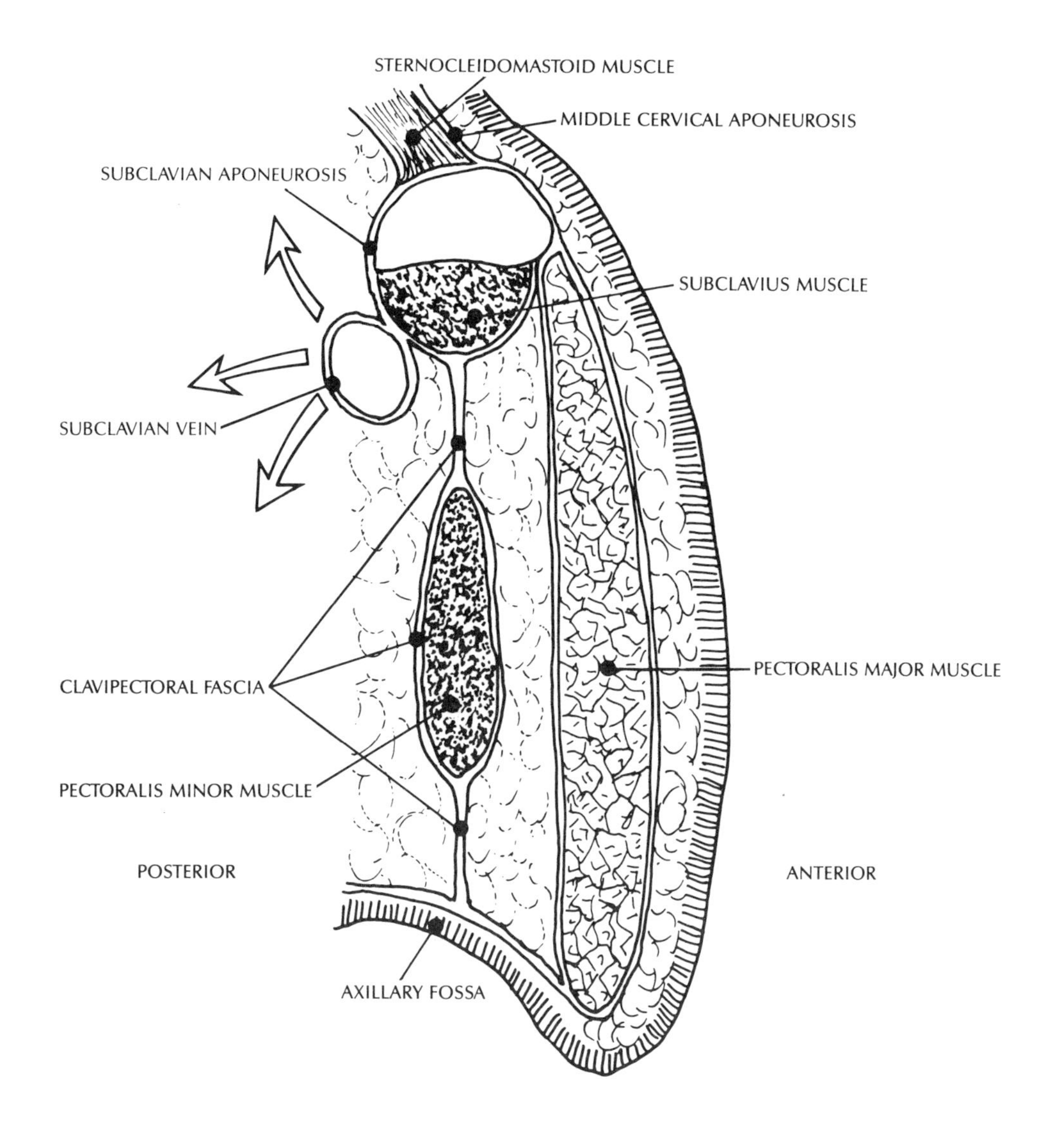

Illustration 2-13
Subclavian Aponeurosis (after Testut & Jacob)

The subclavian aponeurosis is continuous with the middle cervical aponeurosis above, and the clavipectoral fascia below. Because of the fibers it shares with the former, the subclavian aponeurosis also plays a role in venolymphatic circulation.

CLAVIPECTORAL FASCIA

This covers an area bounded generally by the clavicle, coracoid process, and axilla (Illustration 2-14). It inserts superiorly on the sheath of the subclavius muscle and on the coracoid. Lower down, it covers the clavipectoral triangle, connecting the subclavius and pectoralis minor muscles. It surrounds the latter and merges with its aponeurosis, the skin of the axillary fossa, and the brachial aponeurosis at the level of the coraco-

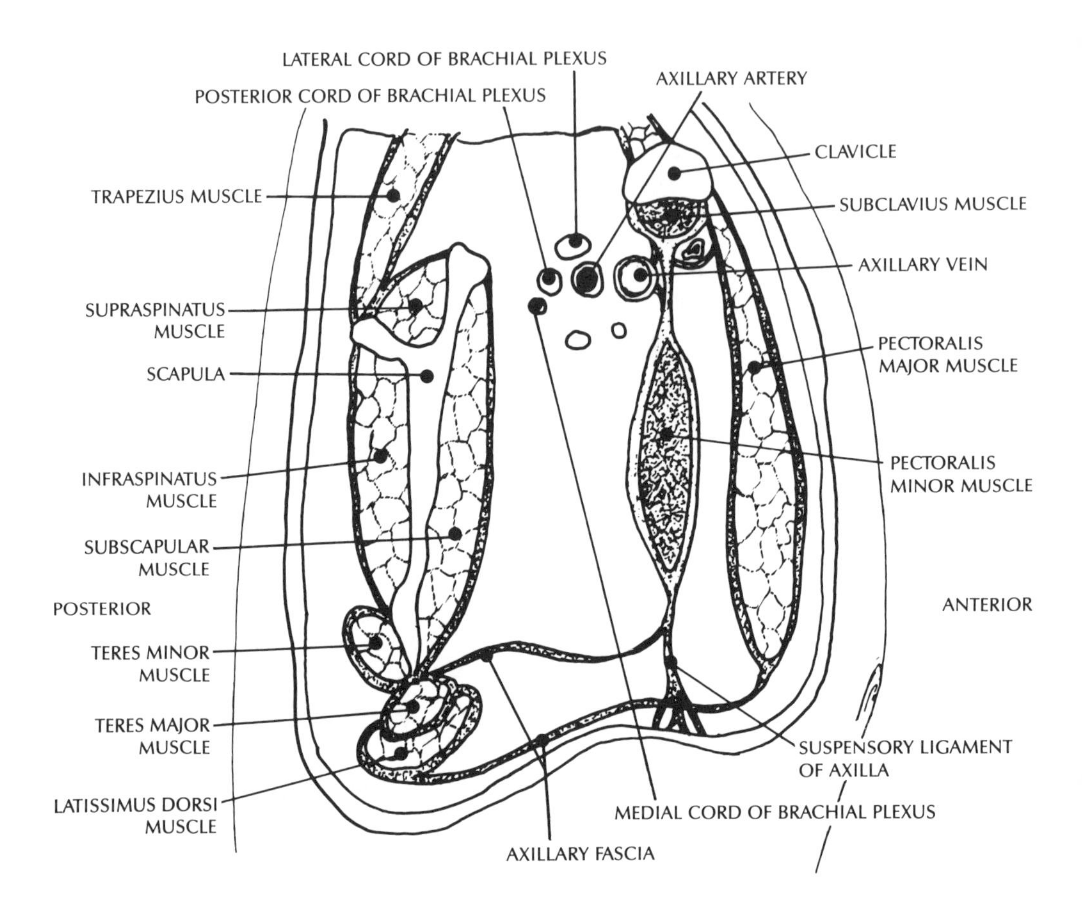

Illustration 2-14
Clavipectoral Fascia (after Charpy & Nicolas)

brachialis muscle and short head of the biceps brachii. At this point it turns into the suspensory ligament of the axilla. Any time the middle cervical aponeurosis requires treatment, you should search for fibrosis or adhesions of the clavipectoral fascia, which is continuous with it via the subclavian aponeurosis. The clavipectoral fascia can be used to stretch the middle cervical aponeurosis, and to work on the subclavius muscle.

The clavipectoral fascia joins the cervical spine and thorax to the arm. As discussed later, the arm has to be placed in proper position for its stretching so that the coracobrachialis and biceps muscles are under tension. This fascia is often reinforced by the medial coracoclavicular ligament, whose mobility should be checked when there are problems with the fascia.

PLEURA

At the beginning of our dissection studies, this was certainly the fascia which interested us the most. We have discussed its role as a pressure equalizer in our previous books, and shall focus here on its parietal layer (and particularly its attachments) because of its osteopathic importance. The parietal layer lines the entire thoracic cavity. This thin tissue layer adheres at the bottom to the diaphragm.

Pleural restrictions are common because of the many problems which can affect the lungs. These include pollution, tuberculosis, various lung diseases, pleurisy, pneumothorax, trauma to the ribs, and possibly the effects of certain vaccinations (as discussed earlier).

The pleura is probably the structure most affected by the twenty-four thousand daily diaphragmatic movements, particularly in its superior attachments. In this area the gradients and effects of myofascial tensions and changes in pressure are considerable.

Anteriorly and laterally, the parietal pleura lines the sternocostal wall. It is very tough here, and its deeper part is continuous with the endothoracic fascia. This can result in compression of adjacent subpleural tissues. The costal pleura is fairly easy to detach and may develop adhesions in association with certain pleural disorders. It is thick and fibrous and can fix part of the lung, or even the rib cage. The mediastinal pleura are not discussed here because we have not found any use for them in osteopathic manipulations.

Suspensory Apparatus

The parietal pleura is attached to a connective tissue dome which serves as an intermediary to the skeleton. This dome consists of myofascial fibers and ligaments, e.g., the pleurovertebral and costopleural ligaments and some fibers of the scalenus minimus muscle, if present (Illustration 2-15).

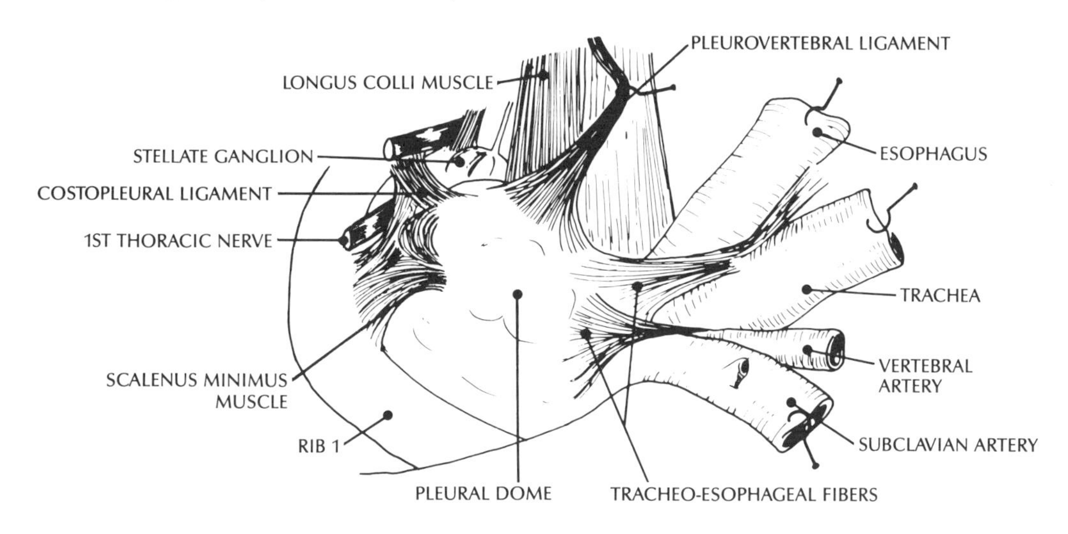

Illustration 2-15
Suspensory Apparatus of the Pleura and the Pleural Dome
(after Charpy & Nicolas)

The *scalenus minimus muscle* seems to occur in about 35% to 65% of the population. When missing, it is often replaced by fibrous tissue containing numerous contractile fibers. It typically originates on the pleural dome, runs superiorly along the superior edge of rib 1, against the anterior scalene, and inserts on the transverse processes of C6-C7.

The *transverse cupular ligament* is better developed when the scalenus minimus muscle is absent, since it has essentially the same course. It is also known as the suprapleural membrane.

The *costopleural ligament* consists of thick connective fibers which connect the pleural dome to the neck of rib 1. From here the ligament runs along the anterior edge of rib 1 to end next to the anterior scalene. It is bound quite tightly to the pleura.

At this point it is appropriate to reemphasize the importance of the five important fibromuscular attachments around the scalene tubercle. These are the anterior scalene muscle, costopleural ligament, scalenus minimus muscle, an expansion of the deep cervical aponeurosis, and some of the fibers of the pleural dome.

The fascial extensions of the middle and deep cervical aponeuroses are in contact with the pleura. They help attach it to the cervical spine, neck of rib 1, and to organs such as the esophagus and trachea.

These fasciae are divided into two principal parts—the first running from C4-C7 to the pleural dome, the second detaching itself from the middle cervical aponeurosis and running to the inferior part of the dome.

Relationships: The pleural suspensory apparatus extends as far as 2-3cm above the medial extremity of the clavicle. From front to back, this apparatus relates to the internal thoracic artery and vein, subclavian artery and vein, origins of the vertebral and superior intercostal arteries, stellate ganglion, and the most inferior branches of the brachial plexus.

There is a cavity medial to the costopleural ligament, and lateral to the pleurovertebral ligament. The bottom of the longus colli muscle, and the stellate ganglion and superior intercostal artery, are located here. Between the ligaments and rib 1 is the fissure through which the first thoracic nerve passes.

There is an aponeurotic extension (sometimes known as the scalenopleural ligament) which runs from the medial sheath of the anterior scalene to the anterior pleural dome. The subclavian nerve runs along the anterior side of this ligament.

Osteopathic remarks: The cervicopleural attachments are one of the most interesting areas of the body. The continuously mobile pleura needs to be upheld. Pleuropulmonary mobility is obviously dependent on this superior attachment. It is somewhat paradoxical that the cervical spine is much more mobile than the thorax, but at the same time serves as a superior fixed point for the pleural system.

The suspensory attachments of the pleura and pericardium are inserted around the spinal column, particularly on the deep cervical aponeurosis covering C7 and T1. Some authors refer to a "cervicothoracic diaphragm" sprinkled with openings or loosely-organized tissue through which pass the pleura, thymus, large vessels, trachea, and esophagus. The peripheral partition of this "diaphragm" consists of the juxtaposition of connective tissue structures such as the sternal and clavicular insertions of the middle cervical aponeurosis anteriorly, the vascular sheaths laterally, and the visceral sheaths and fibromuscular pleural apparatus posteriorly.

We believe that degenerative problems of the lower cervical spine cannot be explained entirely in terms of mobility disorders of the cervical vertebrae, or the gravitational lines of the spine. Pleuropulmonary tension, a permanent and active force, must also be involved. During our work in pulmonary departments of hospitals, we were struck by how often radiology or dissection demonstrated overworked or eroded lower cervical vertebrae. Abnormal tension of the accessory inhalatory muscles was a frequent cause, although this phenomenon seems to occur particularly in association with thickening and fibrosis of the pleura.

In view of the relationships between the pleural attachments and neurovascular system, it is easy to imagine the disorders which can arise in this strategic area, and their effects on nearby organs.

Recesses

In osteopathy, the recesses are particularly relevant when there are sequelae to pleural pathologies. These lines of pleural reflection can then affect many other pleuropulmonary and sternocostal structures. This is not surprising in view of the interchange of fibers between the subcostal and internal intercostal muscles and the pleura (Illustration 2-16). In this section, we will describe specific recesses and techniques which can be applied to them.

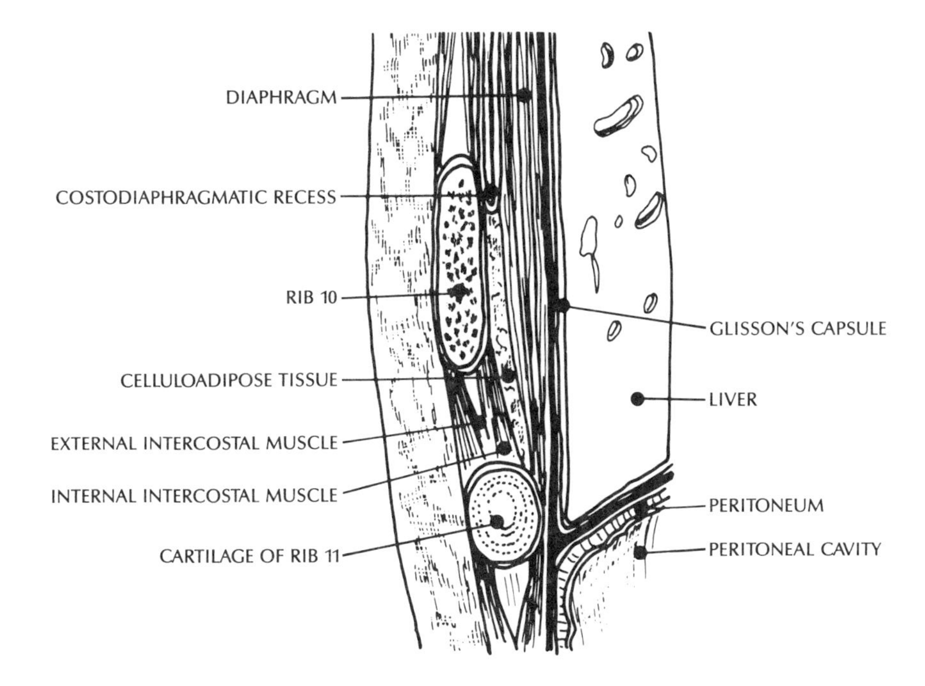

Illustration 2-16
Right Costodiaphragmatic Recess (after Testut & Jacob)

The right and left *costomediastinal recesses* delineate between them an hourglass-shaped surface, like two triangles overlapping at the tips. The upper triangle contains the thymus (or, in adults, the adipose mass which replaces it), while the lower triangle corresponds to the pericardium, directly in contact with the sternocostal plane. The exact location of these recesses varies considerably, but in general the tips of the two triangles overlap around the third and fourth sternocostal joints, slightly to the left of the midline. Since the costomediastinal recesses adhere to the transversus thoracis muscle, stretching of this muscle has an effect on pleural restrictions.

Certain important zones of insertion are helpful in placing your hands for stretching the right costomediastinal recess. These are the right sternoclavicular and second and seventh sternochondral joints. The fourth sternochondral joint is also used because of its relationship with the right horizontal fissure (described later). The left costomediastinal recess is stretched by placing your hands on the left sternoclavicular and fourth and sixth left sternochondral joints.

The insertions of the costodiaphragmatic recesses are approximately the same on the left and right sides. Anterior landmarks for locating this recess are the seventh sternochondral joint, and costal cartilages 8-10. Inferolaterally it is 2-3cm from the anterior extremity of rib 11, and superolaterally it is bounded by rib 9. Posteriorly, this recess extends 1-1.5cm behind rib 12 (we use this fact to fix the pleura during manipulations). Superficially, it contacts the upper part of rib 10.

PERICARDIUM

This very tough fibrous/serous sac is about 14cm long and 10cm wide at the bottom. The sternum is separated from the fibrous pericardial sac by loose connective tissue which condenses at the top and bottom to form the superior and inferior sternopericardial ligaments. At around eight years of age, the thymus degenerates into a fibrous/adipose mass which separates the pericardium from the sternum between ribs 1 and 3. Our dissections have verified that the thymus is progressively transformed into pericardial ligaments, as suggested by various authors.

Posteriorly, the pericardium relates to the organs contained in the posterior mediastinum, from the level of T4 to T8. In a vertical position, T8 goes slightly above the heart; this vertebra corresponds with the diaphragmatic wall and apex of the heart. Inferiorly, the pericardium is attached to the central tendon of the diaphragm. Medially, it is closely linked to the esophagus by connective tissue tracts. Because of this relationship, it is often difficult to differentiate between esophagitis, esophageal spasm, and cardiac problems (see Chapter 4).

The topography of the pericardium will be discussed later in relation to the heart.

Ligaments

The erect position of humans necessitates that the pericardium have strong superior attachments; otherwise the heart would be compressed in certain positions. According to Pierre Mercier, the general axis of the thorax goes through the anterior part of the heart, which would explain why this organ is little implicated in thoracic movements. The pericardium also serves as a means of fixation for the center of the diaphragm, preventing excessive stretching of the vessels during certain movements. The pericardium is attached to the sternum and spinal column by various ligaments, as described below. There are also phrenopericardial ligaments, which do not need to be described here.

The *superior sternopericardial ligament* (sometimes called the sternocostopericardial ligament) is triangular and inserted on the manubrium and first sternocostal joint. As the thymus degenerates, this ligament seems to replace it. One group of fibers runs to the manubrium and another to the middle cervical aponeurosis. This ligament helps suspend the pericardium in the vertical and supine positions.

The *inferior sternopericardial ligament* (sometimes called the xiphopericardial ligament) is also roughly triangular in shape. It originates at the bottom of the xiphoid process, exchanges several fibers with the diaphragm, and inserts into the middle part of the diaphragm. It is less resistant than its superior counterpart, and helps suspend the heart in the supine position.

The *vertebropericardial ligaments* insert into a thickened portion of the deep cervical aponeurosis between C4 and T4. Some of the fibers run anteriorly to form aponeurotic sheaths for the aorta and large vessels at the base of the neck. These ligaments are better developed on the left side. This may help explain the fact that with certain pathologies of the heart, vertebropericardial restrictions are more predominant on the left, as we have observed in clinical practice.

The ligaments described above play an important role as attachments of the pericardium, which reinforces our emphasis on the cervicothoracic junction. Some osteopaths state that C7/T1 is often fixed because of its intense energetic effect on the body (which in turn is related to function of the thyroid, parathyroids, etc.) We prefer to concentrate on the anatomy of this region before putting too much emphasis on its energetic role. A good understanding of the complex anatomy around C7/T1 is more than sufficient to explain the impressive results often obtained from manipulation in this area.

Visceral System

LUNGS

We have tried many techniques for treatment of the lungs, but only those applied to the pleural attachments and the fissures (see below) gave noteworthy results. Rather than describe the lungs in exhaustive detail, we will therefore focus on (and to a degree simplify) the localization of these fissures (Illustrations 2-17 and 2-18).

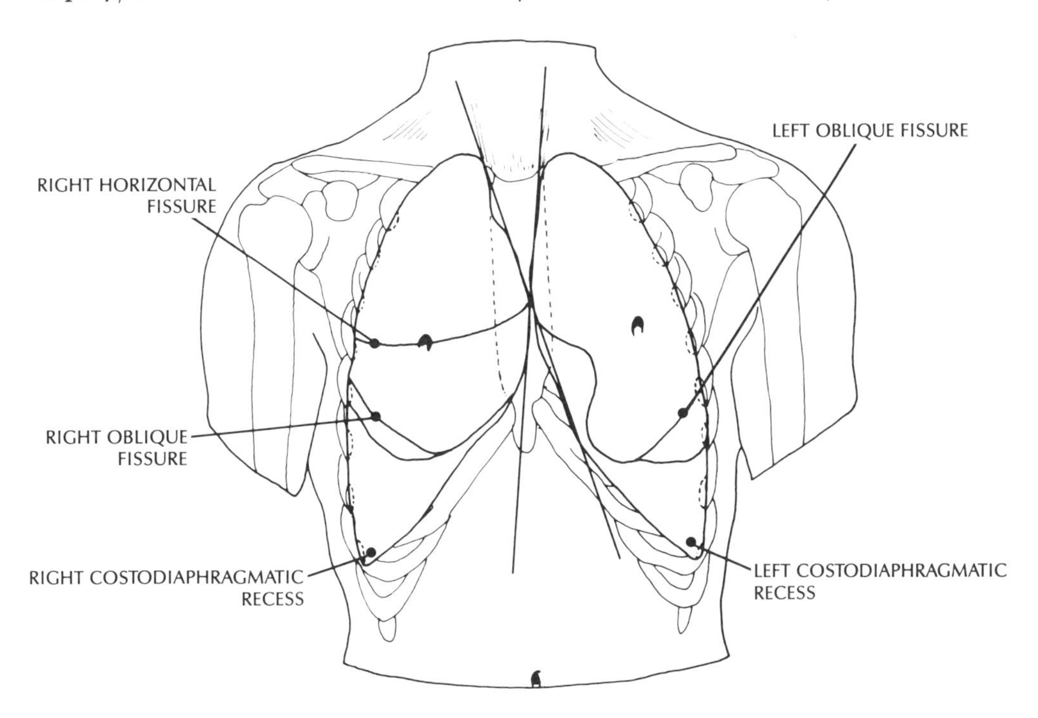

Illustration 2-17
Recessess and Fissures: Anterior View (after Testut & Jacob)

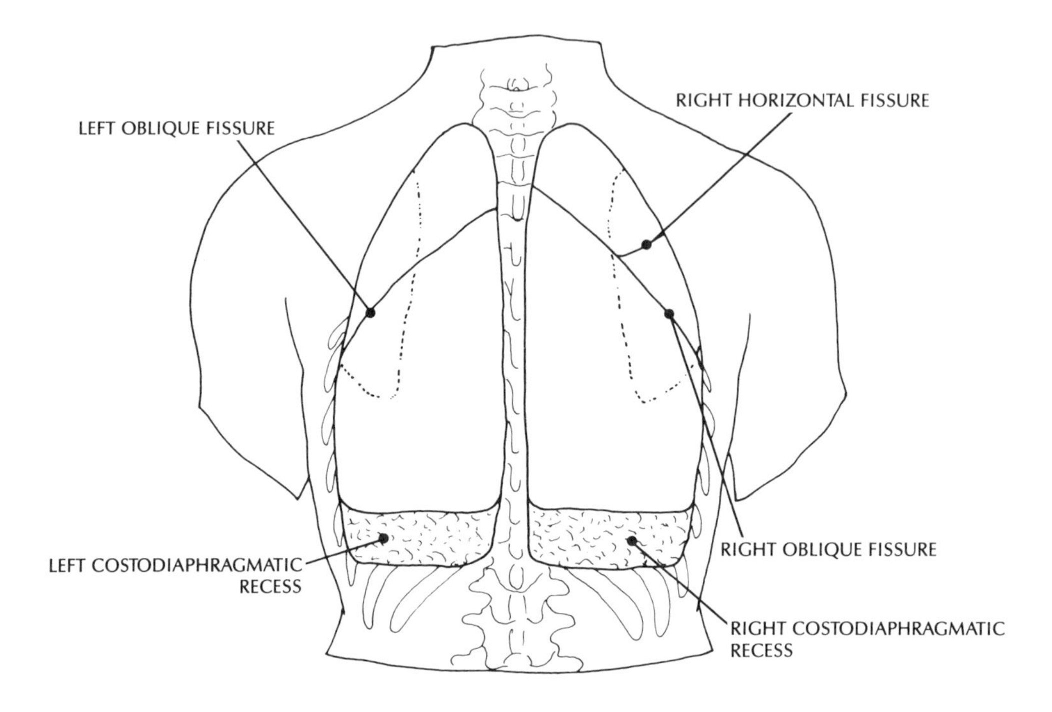

Illustration 2-18
Recessess and Fissures: Posterior View (after Charpy & Nicolas)

Fissures

The *left oblique fissure* begins posterosuperiorly near the fourth costovertebral joint and ends anteroinferiorly near the sixth sternochondral joint, crossing rib 5 at an oblique angle. For manipulation, note that it has close relationships anteriorly with ribs 5-6, and posteriorly with ribs 4-5.

The *right oblique fissure* begins posterosuperiorly near the third costovertebral joint and ends anteroinferiorly near the sixth rib. For manipulation, note that it has close relationships anteriorly with rib 6, and posteriorly with ribs 3, 4, 5, and 6 (medially to laterally).

The *horizontal fissure* separates itself posteriorly from the oblique fissure at the medial scapula between ribs 4 and 5, and ends anteriorly just below the third sternochondral joint. We are most interested in the anterior part because of its close relationship with the third sternochondral joint and rib 4.

THYMUS

We know very little about this gland. Some osteopaths apply pumping techniques to it, but these have not been shown to have any noteworthy effect. Like the spleen, the thymus cannot be palpated unless there is significant pathology, and manipulation remains mostly theoretical. We have never been able to feel it with our listening techniques, except in cases of Hodgkin's disease.

The thymus is found at the top of the anterior mediastinum and follows respiratory movements. As mentioned above, it becomes transformed in adulthood into the superior sternopericardial ligament. In early childhood there is a cervical portion, but this progressively turns into a sort of thyrothymic ligament. The upper limit of the thymus is the sternal notch; the lower limit is usually found around the third and fourth intercostal spaces. The posteroinferior side relates to the pericardium, and the lateral sides to the mediastinal pleura and lungs. The thymus is surrounded by a fibrous capsule which attaches it to the pericardium and middle cervical aponeurosis.

HEART

Osteopathic manipulation is unable to treat pathologies of the cardiac muscle itself. We have had some success in alleviating symptoms in cases of angina and coronary artery disease, but have been unable to document physiological changes in these patients. Instead of discussing the heart itself, we will focus on the pericardium and coronary arteries. In clinical practice, the surface projection of the pericardium can be confused with that of the heart.

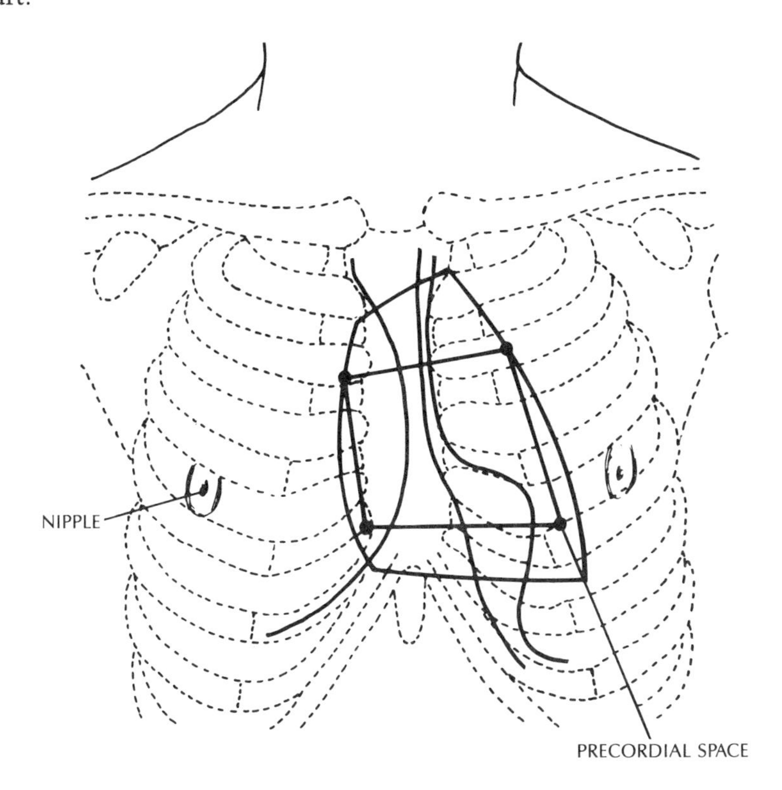

Illustration 2-19
Anterior Topography of the Pericardium (after Testut & Jacob)

Pericardium

Most pericardial techniques are carried out from the front. Important reference points are shown in Illustration 2-19. The upper boundary of the pericardium is an imaginary plane joining the first left to the second right sternochondral joint; the lower boundary is a plane joining the sixth right sternochondral joint to the sixth left intercostal space, 6-8cm from the edge of the sternum (this plane passes through the base of the body of the sternum).

Only a small part of the pericardium is in direct contact with the sternochondral wall; the rest is covered by the costomediastinal recess. Actually, the mediastinal pleura is connected to the pericardium via an adipose tissue layer, rather than directly. The outer portion of the pericardium is roughly triangular, with the base uniting the two sixth sternochondral joints, the summit near the third left sternochondral joint, and the sides following the costomediastinal recesses.

Only the left side of the pericardium is accessible to manipulation or listening techniques, since the right side is hidden behind the sternum. This accessible portion is also roughly triangular, with the summit close to the fourth left sternochondral, the base near the sixth and seventh left sternochondral joints, the right side on the left edge of the sternum, and the left side at the left costomediastinal recess.

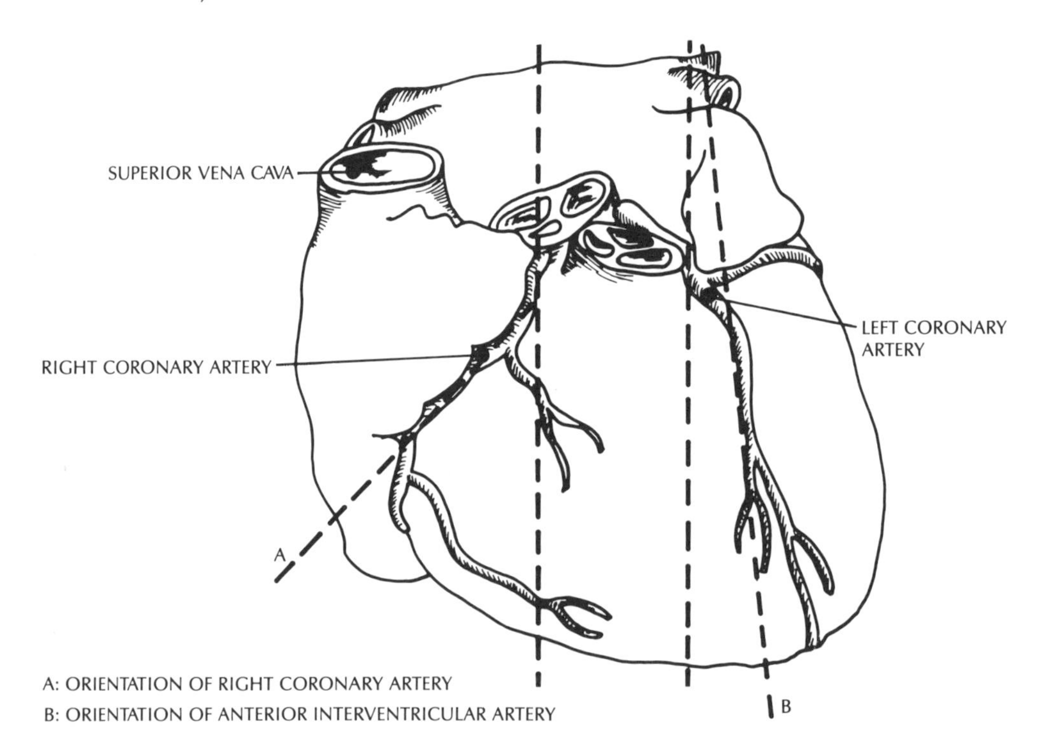

Illustration 2-20
Orientation of the Coronary Arteries (after Khale)

Coronary Arteries

Orientation of the coronary arteries is shown in Illustration 2-20. The right coronary artery runs downward and to the right, making an angle of approximately 40 degrees with the midline. This angle begins nearly at the third left sternochondral joint, and descends along the left atrioventricular sulcus. The left coronary artery, after branching off the left aorta, divides quickly into the circumflex artery and an anterior interventricular artery (also known as the left anterior descending artery), which travels in the anterior interventricular sulcus. The orientation of the anterior interventricular artery forms an angle of approximately 20 degrees with the midline, beginning near the third sternochondral joint.

Vascular System

As mentioned in Chapter 1, mechanical restrictions of the thoracic inlet can have a variety of vascular consequences. Manipulation of the vertebral column and viscera can be useless if one neglects to release all the perivascular tissues. The subclavian artery and vein are of particular interest. In this section, we will describe some aspects of vascular topography relevant to osteopathic diagnosis and treatment.

AORTA

The ascending aorta is located behind the middle of the manubrium, its inferior extremity being at the level of the line which joins the third sternochondrals. The aorta reaches the first left sternochondral joint at its highest point, and then bends backwards and to the left. In adults, its highest point is approximately 2cm above the sternal notch.

BRACHIOCEPHALIC VESSELS

The *brachiocephalic artery* is only found on the right. Its sternal projection is on the midline, and limited inferiorly by the line connecting the two first sternochondral joints. The *brachiocephalic veins* result from the union of the subclavian and internal jugular veins, and are surrounded by fibrous tracts arising from the middle cervical aponeurosis. The right vein lies below the right sternoclavicular and first right sternochondral joints. The left vein corresponds to the inferior left sternoclavicular joint and to a line on the sternum leading from this joint to the medial part of the first right intercostal space.

SUBCLAVIAN ARTERIES AND THEIR BRANCHES

A good understanding of the complicated vascular anatomy in the supraclavicular region (Illustration 2-21) requires a lot of work, but is well worthwhile.

The subclavian arteries are of great clinical importance. They are frequently compressed by bony or firm neighboring structures of the thoracic inlet, with a variety of resulting clinical symptoms. The right and left subclavians arise from the brachiocephalic artery and aortic arch respectively; they are 6cm and 8cm long respectively, with a diameter of about 8mm, and show a narrowing in the middle. The right is more anterior than the left.

The subclavian arteries have many branches, which explains why their compression can have such a variety of effects. Among these branches are the vertebral arteries, internal thoracic arteries (which anastomose with the epigastric), thyrocervical trunk (which in turn gives rise to the inferior thyroid and transverse cervical arteries), and costocervical trunk (which gives rise to the first intercostal and deep cervical arteries).

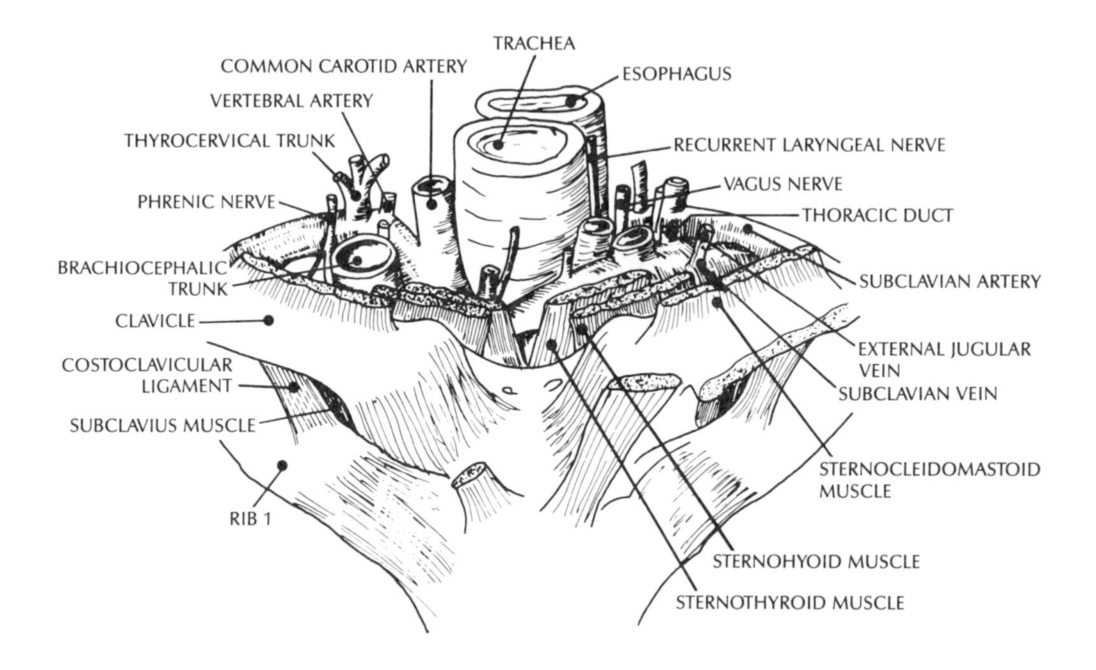

Illustration 2-21
Supraclavicular Vascular Anatomy (after Charpy & Nicolas)

The *right subclavian artery* arises from the brachiocephalic artery at the level of the right sternoclavicular joint (Illustration 2-22). Anteriorly, it is deep to the subcutaneous tissue, platysma muscle, clavicle, inferior insertions of the sternocleidomastoid, sternohyoid, and sternothyroid muscles. Below the muscles, there is an area sometimes called the venous angle or Pirogoff's angle where the subclavian vein, jugular veins, vertebral vein, and large lymphatic ducts converge. Behind the venous angle, three nerves cross over the anterior side of the right subclavian: the phrenic laterally, a large branch of the sympathetic trunk medially, and, between the two, the vagus. The phrenic nerve sends out a recurrent fiber which passes underneath to join the stellate ganglion. The vagus nerve crosses over the artery near its origin, slightly inside the sternoclavicular joint, and sends out a recurrent branch at this point. Because of the close relationship between the artery and these nerves, compression of the former typically affects the latter also, further increasing the number of nonspecific symptoms that can arise from compression of the thoracic inlet. Posteriorly, the right subclavian is separated from the transverse process of C7 by the stellate ganglion, first thoracic root, and pleural transversus muscle; any of these structures can be affected by fibrosis of the cervicopleural attachments. Finally, the pleura is immediately inferior to the right subclavian, so that there is interdependence between these two structures.

The *left subclavian artery*, which is intrathoracic and arises from the left side of the aortic arch, is often compressed by pleural scars associated with left pleuropulmonary pathologies, as we have observed in dissections. This artery branches off the aorta 3cm lateral to the medial extremity of the left clavicle. Anteriorly, it contacts the carotid artery and the origin of the left brachiocephalic vein, which separates it from the sternum.

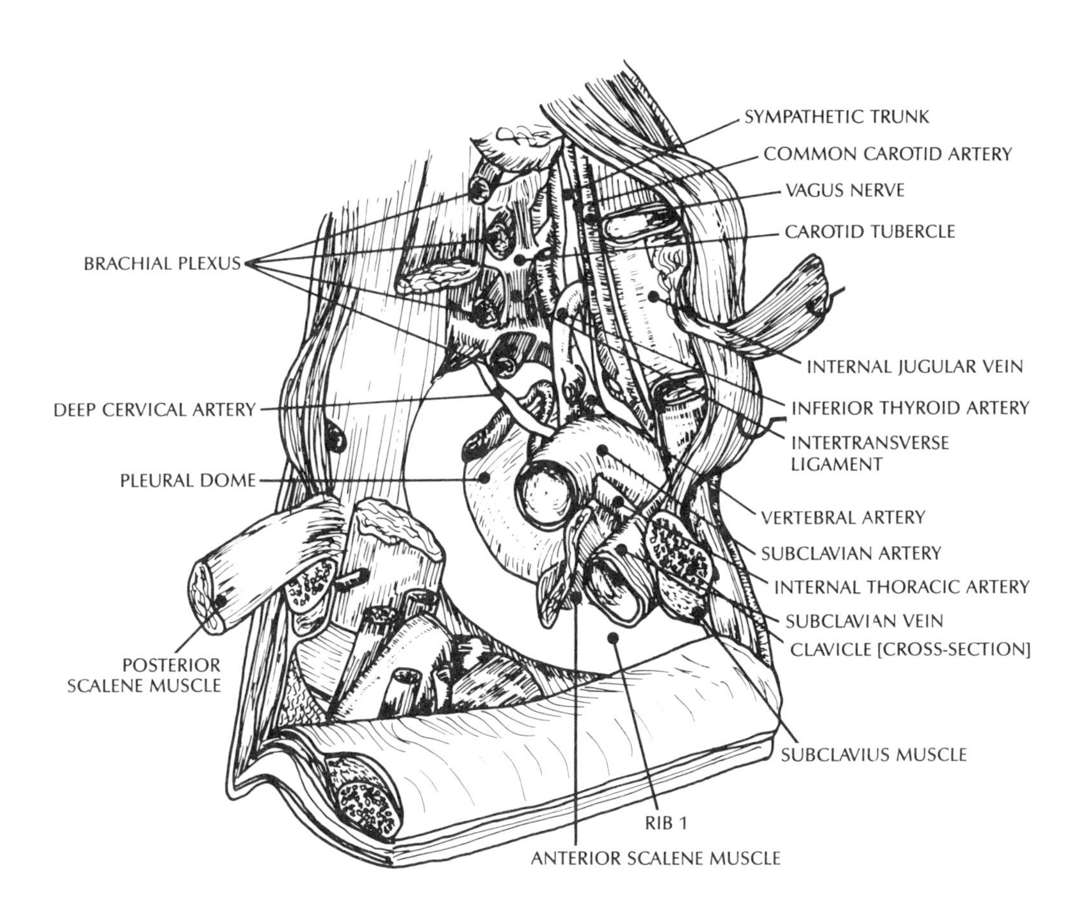

Illustration 2-22
Relationships of the Right Subclavian Artery

Posteriorly, it is separated from the thoracic spine by the longus colli muscle. It relates to the trachea, esophagus, recurrent laryngeal nerve, and lymphatic nodes medially, and to the mediastinal pleura laterally. The left subclavian can be divided into intrascalenic, interscalenic, and extrascalenic portions, the latter being of greatest interest in regard to the cervicothoracic junction. This extrascalenic portion is located in the subclavian fossa, where it is accessible to our techniques, but also vulnerable to trauma (Illustration 2-23). It rests on the first rib, outside and behind the scalene tubercle, which is the insertion site for the anterior scalene, scalenus minimus, costopleural ligament, and extensions of the deep cervical aponeurosis, subclavian aponeurosis, and pleural dome. This tubercle can be palpated approximately 1.5cm medial to the middle of the clavicle, directing the finger posteroinferiorly. Superiorly and posteriorly, the extrascalenic portion of the left subclavian relates to the brachial plexus. Anteriorly, it relates to the subclavian vein, platysma muscle, subcutaneous tissue, superficial cervical aponeuroses, and omohyoid muscle.

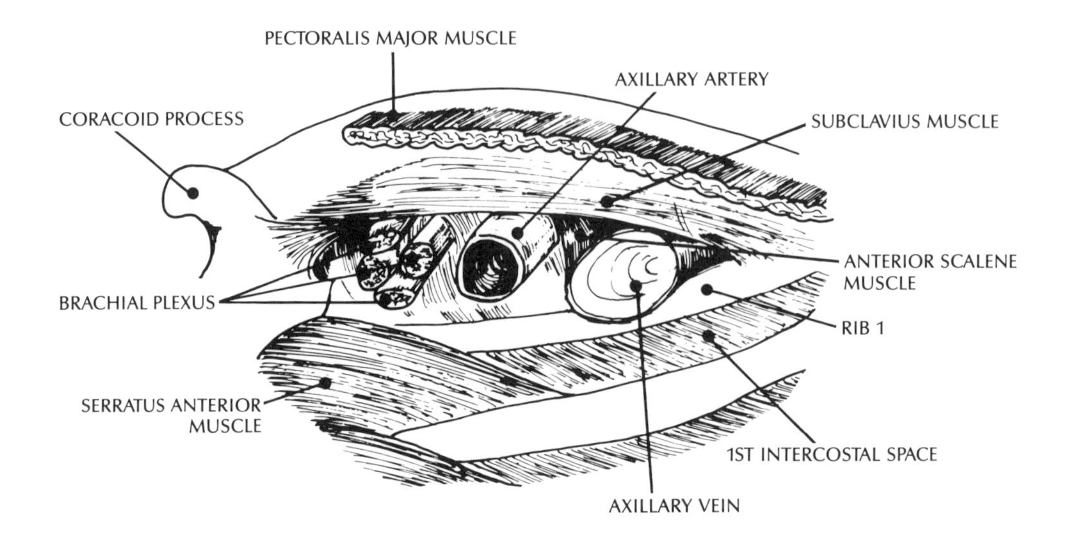

Illustration 2-23
Relationships Between the Subclavian Vessels and the First Rib (after Testut & Jacob)

VERTEBRAL AND BASILAR ARTERIES

We must digress briefly from our focus on the thorax to discuss these arteries of the skull, which arise from the subclavian artery and are functionally related to it.

Each vertebral artery branches off from the subclavian in front of the transverse process of C7, between the longus colli and scalene muscles. It runs through the transverse foramina of C6 through C2 and makes its first bend in order to go between the atlas and axis. Posterior to the body of the atlas, it makes a second bend, traverses the dura mater between the posterior arch of the atlas and occipital foramen, and eventually joins with its counterpart on the opposite side to form the basilar artery (Illustration 2-24), which supplies the posterior brain and inner ear.

The initial portion of the vertebral artery, located at the base of the neck, runs posteroinferiorly between the longus colli and anterior scalene muscles. Its anterior aspect relates to the common carotid artery, vertebral vein, cervical sympathetics, and inferior thyroid artery. Posteriorly, the vertebral artery relates to the transverse process of C7, posterior jugular vein, stellate ganglion, cervical spinal nerves 7 and 8, and in some cases thoracic nerve 1. Laterally, it relates to the scalenus minimus muscle, or its counterpart, the transverse cupular ligament. Medially, it relates to the internal jugular, primary carotid, and vagus nerve.

The vertebral artery, internal thoracic artery, costocervical trunk, and thyrocervical trunk all begin inside the medial edge of the anterior scalene. Since these vessels are densely packed (there is as little as 25mm between the vertebral artery and thyrocervical trunk), mechanical compression in this area can produce a variety of symptoms.

The basilar artery, formed by the union of the two vertebral arteries, in turn gives rise to the pontine branches, anterior inferior cerebellar artery, superior cerebellar artery, and posterior cerebral artery. The internal acoustic artery (also known as the

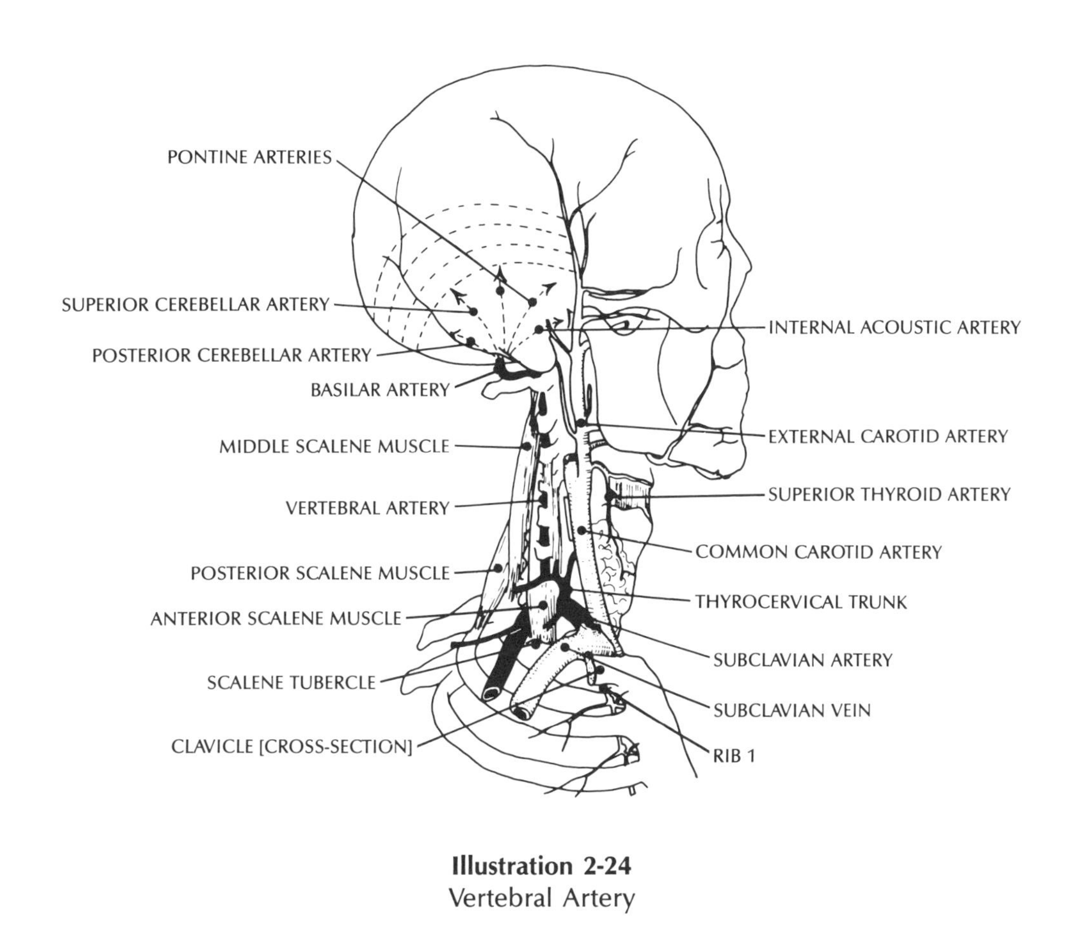

Illustration 2-24
Vertebral Artery

labyrinthine artery) branches off either the basilar artery or anterior inferior cerebellar artery and supplies the organs of the inner ear. This explains the balance problems that are sometimes associated with compression of the subclavian artery.

SUBCLAVIAN VEIN

In diagnosing pathologies of the thoracic inlet, many practitioners consider only arterial function. However, the subclavian vein is in front of the subclavian artery, and our experience indicates that it is the first vessel injured by traumatic or scarring processes of the inlet. As mentioned earlier, this and other veins of the cervicothoracic junction have an "inhalatory emptying" function due to their attachments to various vascular sheaths and aponeuroses. The subclavian vein, located above the clavicle, is partially surrounded by a fascial sheet derived from the subclavian aponeurosis, which attaches it to the superior part of rib 1. The vein moves relatively freely on the rib during inhalation or elevation of the shoulder girdle. It is accessible to us via the cervical, middle, or subclavian aponeuroses.

The subclavian vein forms a right angle at its superolateral junction with the internal jugular. This area, which we mentioned earlier, is called the venous angle since it represents the convergence of the external and anterior jugular veins, vertebral vein, and large lymphatic vessels. The surface projection of the venous angle is at the lateral edge of the clavicular attachment of the sternocleidomastoid.

THORACIC DUCT

This major vessel receives lymphatic fluid from parts of the body below the diaphragm, and the left side of the body above the diaphragm. After ascending from the lower body, it forms a lateral arch at the level of C7 (the arch rises 3-4cm above the clavicle), running anterior to the vertebral artery and vein, sympathetic trunk, and thyrocervical trunk. It also passes anterior to the phrenic nerve and medial border of the anterior scalene (from which it is separated by the deep cervical aponeurosis), and ends at the venous angle, forming an inferior concavity facing the subclavian artery. The presence of this collecting canal explains how major abdominal disorders, particularly malignancies, can produce enlarged lymph nodes in the left supraclavicular fossa. These nodes are called Troisier's nodes.

RIGHT LYMPHATIC DUCT

This vessel receives lymphatic fluid from the upper right quadrant of the body, including the right arm, right side of the head and chest, and part of the convex surface of the liver. It runs along the medial border of the anterior scalene muscle at the base of the neck, and empties into the junction of the internal jugular and right subclavian veins. The presence of right supraclavicular nodes is usually due to pathologies of the thoracic region or, much less commonly, the abdominal region.

Nervous System

The nervous system in the thoracic region, like the circulatory system, is quite complex. In this section, we will present some information pertinent to our later discussion of differential diagnosis and therapeutic manipulation. In Chapter 5, we will describe symptoms caused by compression of the nerves.

STELLATE GANGLION

The cervical sympathetic nervous system extends from the base of the skull to the level of rib 1. It adheres to the middle cervical aponeurosis via a fibrous layer, and lies upon the deep cervical aponeurosis, just inside the anterior tubercles of the transverse processes. It includes three ganglia, of which the stellate ganglion (the most inferior) will be described here. The superior is the largest, but is too far away from the thorax to directly concern us. The middle also lies outside the thorax, and is absent in some individuals.

The stellate ganglion (Illustration 2-25) is close to the neck of rib 1 and the anterior surface of the transverse process of C7, which separates it from the longus colli muscle. It is posterior to the origins of the vertebral and subclavian arteries. It occupies a small niche at the top of the pleura, between the pleurovertebral and costopleural ligaments and the scalenus minimus muscle. Because of a change in direction of the sympathetic trunk at the cervicothoracic junction, the stellate ganglion is oriented along an almost anteroposterior axis.

This ganglion sends gray rami communicantes to cervical nerves 7-8 and thoracic

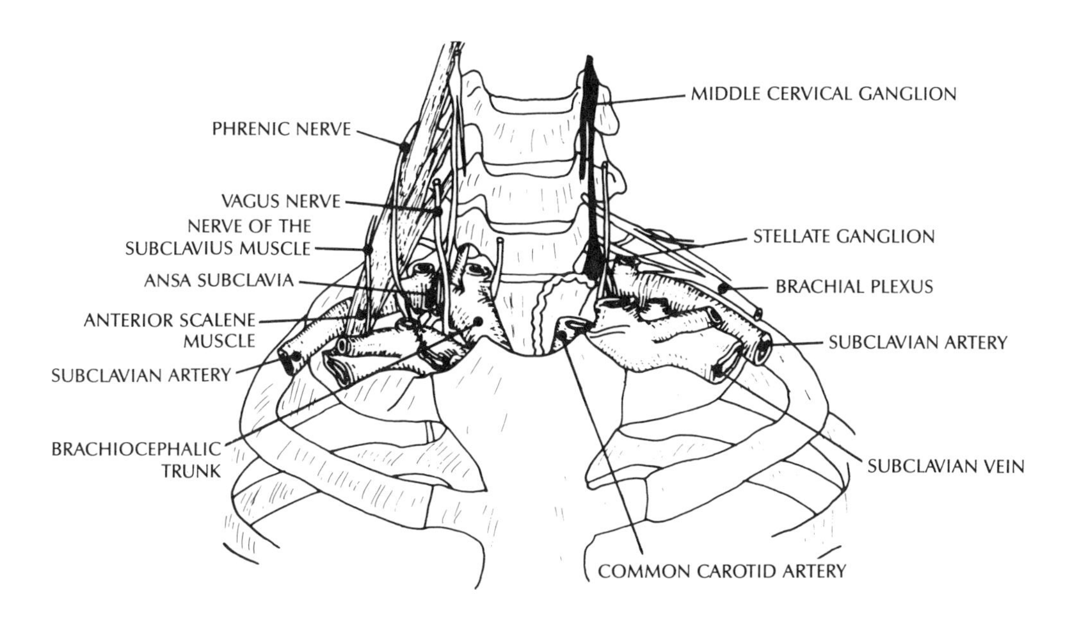

Illustration 2-25
Stellate Ganglion

nerve 1. These include the fibers that innervate the iris, which explains the ipsilateral miosis which appears with restrictions of C7/T1 and rib 1. Superior efferent branches from the ganglion accompany the vertebral artery and its venous network into the intertransverse canal and the skull. Other branches anastomose with the recurrent laryngeal nerve, middle and inferior cardiac nerves, and in some cases the vagus nerve.

FIRST THORACIC GANGLION

The thoracic part of the sympathetic trunk contains a series of ganglia, usually one for each spinal nerve pair. The first thoracic ganglion measures 1-3cm and often merges with the stellate ganglion. It has a half-moon shape, the concave portion being in contact with the posteromedial part of the subclavian artery near the origin of the vertebral artery. This ganglion is close to the articulation between rib 1 and the spinal column. Its primary efferent fibers supply the lungs, thoracic aorta, bones (particularly the vertebrae), trachea, and esophagus.

VAGUS NERVE

This nerve originates in the medulla, passes downward through the jugular foramen and neck (where it is contained in the carotid sheath) and into the thorax. It runs through the posteriorly-directed angle where the internal jugular vein crosses the common carotid artery. The vagus nerve runs anteriorly and laterally to the sympathetic trunk, notably on the anterior side of the transverse processes of C6-C7.

The branches of the vagus are important components of the thoracic inlet (Illustration 2-25). The left branch begins near the origin of the left carotid and subclavian arteries. At the thoracic inlet, it runs posterior to the brachiocephalic vein and medial to the subclavian artery. Within the thorax, it crosses anterior to the aorta and sends a branch to the left recurrent laryngeal nerve. It then adheres to the left anterior part of the esophagus and exits the thorax. The right branch of the vagus runs between the subclavian vein anteriorly and subclavian artery posteriorly. A fiber to the right recurrent laryngeal nerve, which branches off in the neck, is often attached to the pleural dome. This explains some cases of unilateral laryngeal paralysis seen in patients with pleuropulmonary problems. A loop from the right vagus surrounds the subclavian vessels. A similar loop from an anastomotic fiber of the phrenic nerve also surrounds the subclavian vessels on the right. Furthermore, loops of sympathetic nerves from the stellate ganglion (called the ansa subclavia) occur here. For these reasons, disturbance to this area can produce complex and intense neurovascular symptoms.

To locate the vagus nerves, find the two common carotid arteries which, emerging from the thorax, run posterosuperiorly and laterally. Each follows a line from the sternoclavicular joint to the mandibular fossa. As mentioned above, the vagus nerves are contained in the carotid sheaths. Between the head of the sternum and the clavicular origin of the sternocleidomastoid, each carotid is separated from the skin only by the superficial and middle cervical aponeuroses.

Many clinical symptoms relate to specific branches of the vagus nerve; e.g., the meningeal branches are implicated in parietal headaches, and the sensory branches of the external auditory canal can cause otalgia. For more examples, see Chapter 4.

PHRENIC NERVE

This nerve arises mainly from cervical nerve 4, and to a lesser extent 3 and 5. It

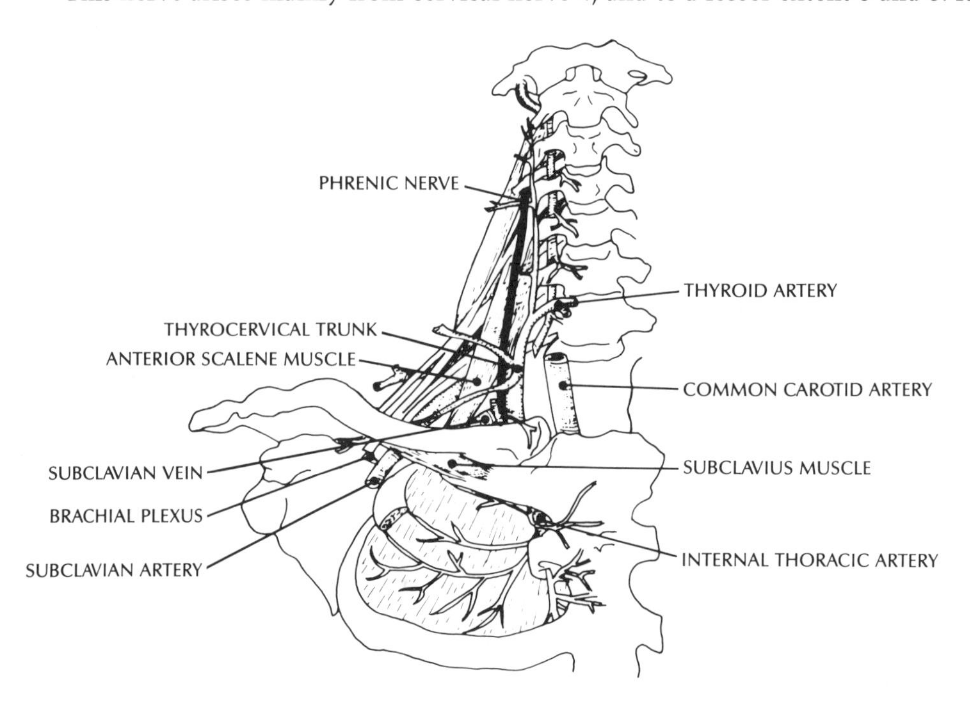

Illustration 2-26
Phrenic Nerve

runs inferiorly, following the anterior side of the anterior scalene, to which it adheres via an aponeurosis (Illustration 2-26). The nerve lies behind the medial extremity of the clavicle, venous angle, thoracic duct on the left, and right lymphatic duct. At the anteroinferior edge of the anterior scalene, the medial edge of the phrenic nerve forms a point within the triangular space which separates the insertion of the two heads of the sternocleidomastoid. This space is called Sedillot's triangle (Illustration 2-27). This point is painful when there is phrenic neuralgia, and is a good trigger point for the thoracic organs and diaphragm.

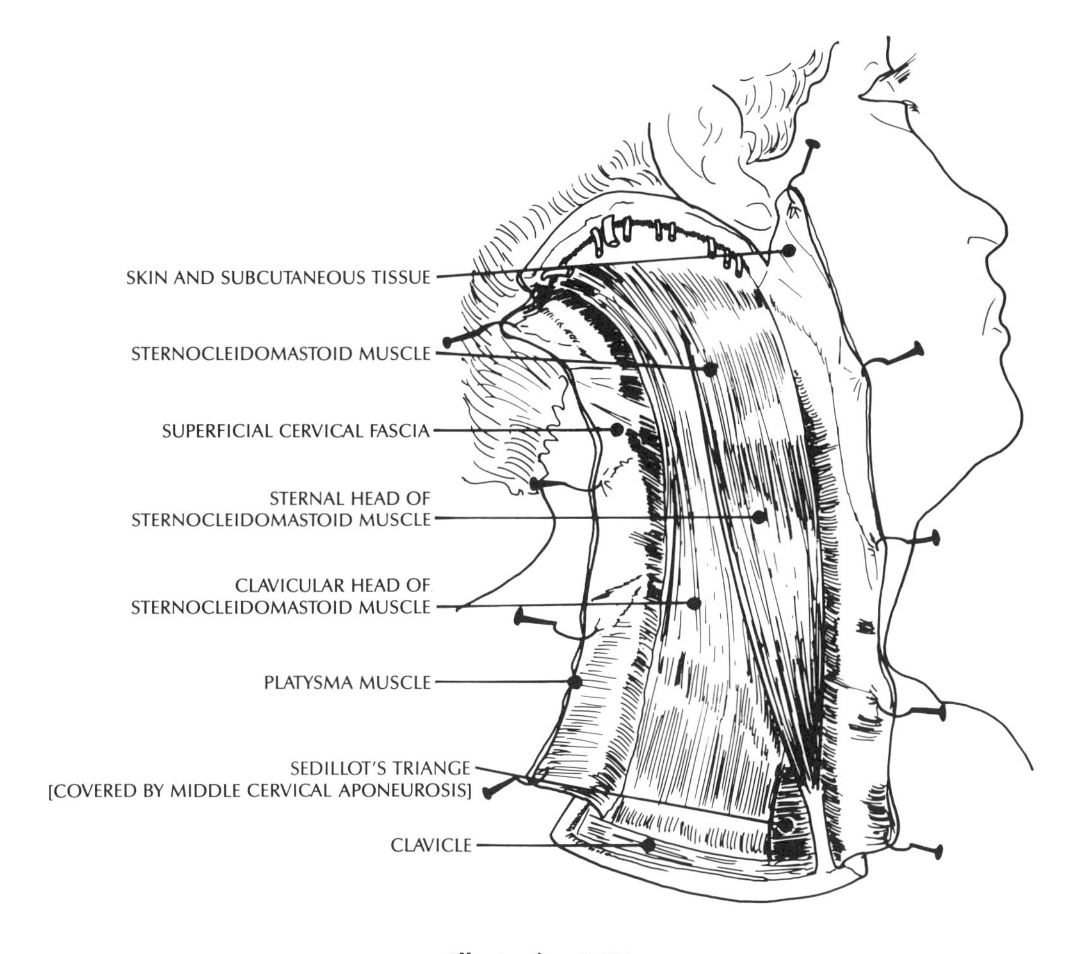

Illustration 2-27
Sedillot's Triangle

CELIAC PLEXUS

The celiac (or solar) plexus is the "abdominal brain" of early anatomists. It consists primarily of a series of anastomosed ganglia and nerves, but also includes blood vessels, nodules of chromaffin matter, adrenal debris, and connective tissue. It is found on the midline of the deep epigastric region, anterior to the aorta and diaphragmatic crura, above the head of the pancreas, and medial to the adrenal capsules. It is bounded above and below by the aortic orifice of the diaphragm and by the renal arteries, respectively. The components of the celiac plexus include the two irregularly shaped celiac ganglia. These lie on the diaphragmatic crura to either side of the aorta, between the origin of the celiac artery and the adrenal glands.

In working on the celiac plexus, we utilize its surface projection, usually located just to the right of the midline, 2-3cm under the seventh right costochondral cartilage. Although it is impossible to palpate the plexus itself, manipulation here produces the most noticeable reactions. On the other hand, the constituent ganglia of this plexus are spread out over a wide area, and it is difficult to demonstrate a right-sided functional predominance (see *Visceral Manipulation II,* p. 28).

CARDIAC PLEXUS

The three sympathetic cardiac nerves anastomose with the cardiac branches of the vagus nerve and the recurrent laryngeal nerve to form the cardiac plexus, which is found around the aortic arch at the fork of the pulmonary artery. The coronary plexuses are derived from the cardiac plexus, as are most of the acceleratory sympathetic cardiac nerves. These relationships explain the functional precordial pain and coronary spasms which are often associated with restrictions of rib 1, particularly on the left.

The surface projection of the cardiac plexus is found to the left of the midline, around the third sternochondral junctions. Our listening techniques often lead us to treat this area, which corresponds anatomically to the superficial cardiac plexus, derived from the superior cardiac fibers of the vagus nerve along with those from the left sympathetic trunk. We obtain our best results here; whether this is because this area is superficial, or functionally more important, is unclear.

Conclusion

Structures of the cervicothoracic junction are anatomically dense and complexly interrelated. Although many osteopaths tend to overemphasize the posterior osteoarticular system, we have observed that abnormal tensions of the anterior soft tissues frequently have major neurovascular effects. We must carefully examine these soft tissues and normalize their functions. Keep in mind that the large vessels are found inside the medial angle of the supraclavicular fossa, where they are closely related to the pleural dome and apex of the lungs. The nerves coming from the brachial plexus are found above and behind the subclavian artery (Illustration 2-28).

Based on these relationships, we can conclude that in general:

- lateral cervicothoracic traumas will have the greatest effect on the nervous system;
- anterior traumas are more likely to affect the vascular system;
- sequelae of pleuropulmonary problems are also likely to affect the vascular system.

In treating thoracic problems, many practitioners focus on arterial function. Although they are relatively difficult to diagnose or treat, we must also pay attention to possible injuries to the venous and lymphatic systems. As mentioned earlier, the

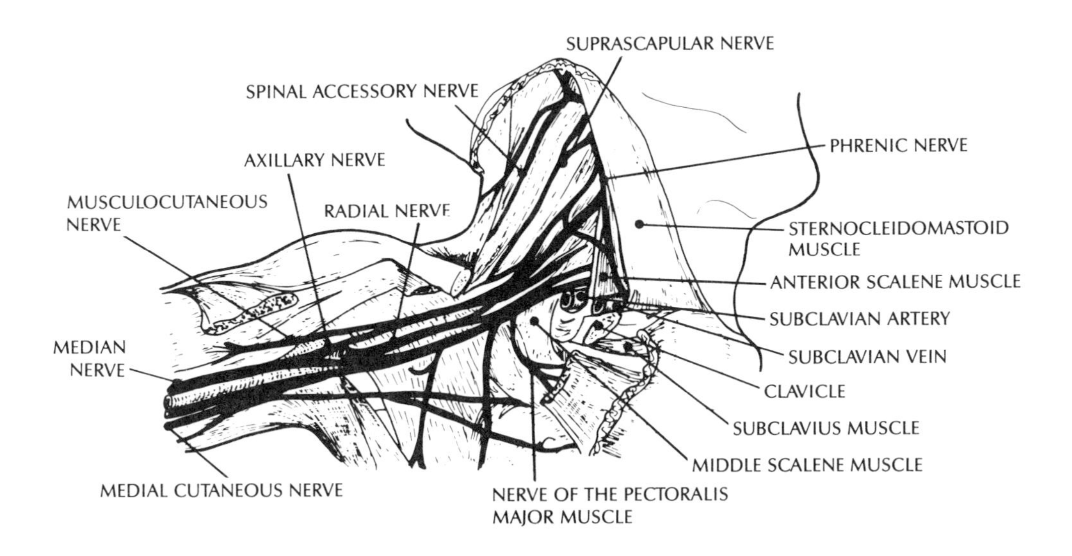

Illustration 2-28
Neurovascular Relationships of the Thoracic Inlet (after Clemente)

subclavian vein is affected before the artery by compression of the thoracic inlet. We would like to emphasize again the essential role of the fasciae (particularly the middle cervical aponeurosis) in venolymphatic circulation of the thoracic inlet.

Finally, we would like to repeat some of the key anatomical points from this chapter that are particularly useful in our work:

- The suspensory system of the pleura is found between rib 1 and the transverse processes of C6-C7.
- The stellate ganglion is on the anterior surface of the transverse process of C7.
- The scalene tubercle is on rib 1, located posteroinferior and 1.5cm medial to the midpoint of the clavicle.
- The inferior insertion of the anterior scalene, on the scalene tubercle, separates the subclavian vein and artery.
- The sternoclavicular joints protect but can also compress the entire cervicothoracic vascular system.
- The phrenic nerve runs through Sedillot's triangle, at the inferior extremity of the anterior scalene, between the two origins of the sternocleidomastoid.
- The pulmonary fissures have a close relationship with ribs 4, 5, and 6.

Chapter Three: Applied Physiology

Table of Contents

CHAPTER THREE

Applied Physiology

The human body contains four major cavities: the skull, thorax, abdomen, and pelvis. Knowledge of the pressure differences existing among these cavities is essential for understanding our techniques. Typical pressures in cm H_20, relative to atmospheric pressure, are: skull +15, thorax −5, abdomen +15, and pelvis +20. Naturally, there are variations among individuals, and among different locations within the same cavity.

The significance of these pressure differences was discussed at length in our previous books. Here, we will focus on some new concepts related to thoracic function.

Pleura

During embryological development, the two pleural cavities become partially separated from the pericardial cavity by membranes. Inferiorly, these three cavities are continuous, which is one reason why we look for peritoneal tension after pleural injuries, and vice versa.

The visceral pleura consists of adherent, thin layers of connective tissue and mesothelium. The connective tissue of the parietal pleura contains many collagenous and elastic fibers, as well as small blood and lymphatic vessels. Both pleurae are highly innervated and can produce painful sensations when irritated. We have seen serious syncopes in association with pleural punctures. As rib restrictions can have a detrimental effect on the pleura, it is particularly important to release these restrictions when treating the pleura.

FORCES

The normal lung increases in volume approximately 200ml when intrapleural pressure falls to 1cm H_20. Therefore, "pulmonary compliance" is about 200 ml/cm H_20.

The lung may be viewed as a bag filled with hundreds of millions of little bubbles which tend to expand or shrink when subjected to variations of pressure.

The visceral pleura is affected by forces of elastic retraction, which tend to pull it back toward the hilum. As lung volume increases, the elastic fibers are progressively stretched and tend to retract with a force proportional to and in the opposite direction from the stretching. Therefore, when treating problems with mobility, one generally works on the movement opposite to the one that is restricted. This means that when working with the contractibility and elasticity of a tissue, it is good to stretch the fibers (i.e., move them in the direction opposite to that in which they contract). In this way, the fibers are "informed" of the possibility of this movement, making it easier for them to perform it on their own.

Because the parietal pleura is closely adherent to the visceral pleura, they are subject to the same forces. The two layers constitute a serous membrane, and are separated by only 2mm of serous fluid (there is only about 50ml of fluid in the virtual space between the two pleurae). Mechanical tension therefore keeps the two layers adherent, without much sliding.

INTRAPLEURAL PRESSURE

Although small, intrapleural pressure can be measured. One reliable method is to have the subject swallow a tube connected to a small balloon which is positioned in the lowest part of the thoracic esophagus, located between the lungs and thoracic walls. Since the esophagus is thin and not resistant to transmission of pressure changes, it is suitable for measurement of intrapleural pressures. However, it is necessary to eliminate or adjust for the effects of deglutition and peristaltic waves. A second method is to introduce a small amount of gas between the two pleurae, thus creating a slight pneumothorax. The pressure measured by a catheter, in this situation, is the resultant of the expansive force of the lung and the retractive force of the chest, i.e., the pressure of the pleural surface, which is subatmospheric.

PRESSURE VARIATIONS

Pleural pressure varies depending on pulmonary volume. It is always negative in the upper part when seated or standing, and in the lower part when lying down. This is one reason why we typically choose the seated position for cervicopleural manipulations and the supine position for mediastinal work. In these positions, the normal tensions of the suspensory muscular/ligamentous system are present and allow restrictions, if present, to be more easily felt. While absolute pressures in the lungs change during respiration, the gradient from bottom to top is essentially constant; pressure at the bottom is 7.5cm H_2O higher than at the top in the standing position (Illustration 3-1). Pleural pressure at the top of the lungs is always negative, varying from −37.5cm H_2O for forced inhalation to −4.5cm H_2O for forced exhalation. Obviously, significant mechanical forces operate at the level of the cervicopleural attachments, and injuries here will interfere with normal pressure changes, thereby affecting pulmonary expansion and circulatory function.

Note that within a single cavity there can be negative pressure at the top and positive pressure at the bottom (Illustration 3-1-C). In our previous books we discussed this phenomenon in the context of the abdominal cavity where, upon deep inhalation,

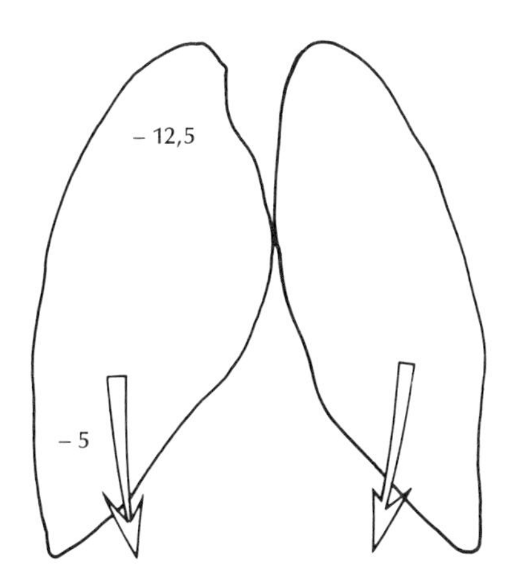

A: DURING NORMAL INHALATION

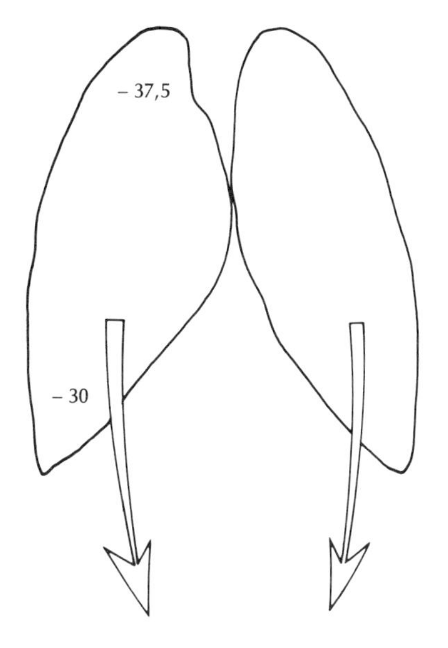

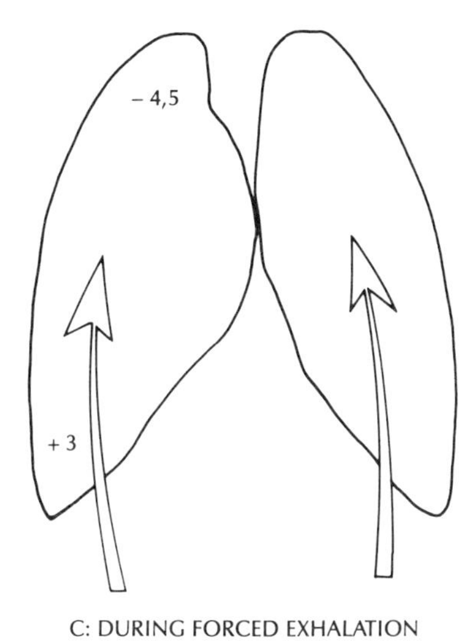

C: DURING FORCED EXHALATION

B: DURING FORCED INHALATION

Illustration 3-1
Pressure Variations

juxtadiaphragmatic intraperitoneal pressure is negative, whereas farther away from the diaphragm it is positive. In the thorax, this type of vertical gradient is controlled by three factors: weight of the lungs, weight of the abdomen, and the chest wall. The effect of the first factor is obvious. The weight of the abdomen has its effect by pulling downward on the diaphragm and pleura. In animal experiments, evisceration diminishes the vertical gradient, but removal of the diaphragm has an even greater effect, possibly because in order to remove the diaphragm it is necessary to resect the viscera attached to it. The effect of the chest wall is demonstrated by the observation that manual compression of the lower part of the chest eliminates the vertical gradient.

The relative contribution of each of these three factors varies from species to species. In most mammals, average contributions are 60% for the abdomen and diaphragm, 25% for chest wall, and 15% for weight of the lungs (Prefaut, 1986). The latter percentage is presumably slightly higher for humans in the vertical position. Clearly, however, the abdominal viscera have a dominant effect upon pleural pressures.

The human body must be viewed in its entirety as an integrated system; i.e., without neglecting the presenting symptom, we must always see beyond it. As we have observed many times in our clinical practice, releasing an abdominal organ can increase pulmonary expansion and thoracic elasticity, while restriction of an abdominal organ can have the opposite effects.

Role of the Myofascial System in Respiration

INHALATION

The external intercostal muscles pull the anterior extremities of the ribs superolaterally, thus increasing the anteroposterior diameter of the thorax. Their contraction also stretches the intercostal spaces and prevents them from being sucked inward during inhalation. In humans, there are five or six particular external intercostals which contract during inhalation. Interestingly, the first seven intercostal spaces have relatively high concentrations of neuromuscular spindles, whereas the diaphragm has few; this may be why we get the best response from treatment of these upper spaces.

The scalenes and sternocleidomastoid are the most important accessory muscles for inhalation. Technically, they are contracted only during deep inhalation. However, we believe that the upward tension they exert during rest helps balance the downward vertical tension exerted on the thorax by the abdomen. Other accessory muscles such as the mylohyoid, digastric, and muscles of the ala nasi assist in inhalation not by increasing thoracic volume, but by reducing resistance to gas flow via correct orientation of respiratory tubes and fasciae.

The middle cervical aponeurosis is an important element in transmission of pressures on a cervicothoracic level. As described earlier, it has attachments to the sternum, clavicles, first ribs, subclavius muscles, and bony or firm landmarks of the thoracic inlet. This aponeurosis allows the inlet to increase in size during inhalation. It also adheres to the connective tissue sheaths of the brachiocephalic veins, subclavian vessels, etc., enabling these large vessels to remain wide open, and in turn permitting the process of inhalation to assist in venolymphatic dynamics.

EXHALATION

According to early physiologists, the abdominal muscles are responsible for exhalation. Actually, this is true only during deep, rapid exhalation, when these muscles help to harmonize and transmit pressures. When exhalation is slightly increased (due to activity), the body reacts by increasing inhalation in order to increase the elastic rebound effect. The internal intercostal muscles lower the ribs, moving them inferomedially, stretch the intercostal spaces to prevent bulging during significant pressure increases (e.g., coughing, sneezing, defecating), and also have a role as pressure regulators. The diaphragm, the primary muscle of inhalation, continues to contract during exhalation, allowing thoracic volume to diminish in a controlled manner. Only near the end of exhalation does the diaphragm completely relax.

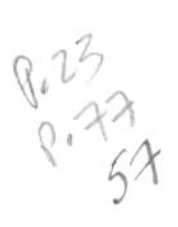

Lung Dynamics

ALVEOLAR VENTILATION

An average of 7-8 liters of air enter the lungs each minute, of which about 5 liters actually enter the alveoli. From this, 300ml oxygen per minute pass through the alveolar and capillary walls to enter the bloodstream, while 250ml $C0_2$ pass in the opposite direction. Thus, about 11,000 liters of air per day enter the lungs, of which less than 5% actually enters the bloodstream.

BLOOD DISTRIBUTION

Besides the heart, the lung is the only organ through which all blood passes. The distribution of blood within the lungs is, naturally, dependent on gravity and body position. In a standing position, there is more blood in the inferior parts of the lungs than in the superior parts. In a subject lying on the back, blood content is similar for superior versus inferior ends of the lung, but greater for posterior versus anterior parts. In the lateral decubitus position, blood content is greater in the inferior part.

DIFFERENTIAL VENTILATION

Gradients of gas flow within the lung are less striking than those of blood flow. Since they have to bear the weight of the entire lung, alveoli in the inferior parts of the lung have a smaller resting volume, are under higher pressure, and presumably are less able to expand. Therefore, total volume of gas moving through the upper parts of the lung is probably higher. On the other hand, the lower parts of the lung may have a greater role in passing oxygen to the arterial circulation simply because they receive a greater supply of blood, as explained above.

Osteopathic Implications

The pleuropulmonary apex is of great interest in osteopathic practice because of various mechanical tensions coexisting in this area. Restrictions of the pleural suspensory system (see Chapter 2) can obviously affect interactions of pressures within the pleuropulmonary system. Many physiological phenomena are dependent on proper pressure interactions, including:

- visceral support and cohesion,
- balanced myofascial tensions,
- proper circulation of blood, lymph, extracellular fluid, and cerebrospinal fluid,
- cardiac output,
- pulmonary ventilation,

- alveolar ventilation,
- esophageal transit.

On the other hand, the inferior parts of the lungs are important in terms of respiratory/circulatory gas exchange, as mentioned above. Aside from major pleural disorders, mechanical problems seem to be less significant in this area.

Chapter Four:

Pathology

Table of Contents

CHAPTER FOUR

Pathology

Differential Diagnosis

Interpretation of chest pain and related symptoms presents some unique difficulties. Here, in contrast to the abdomen, we are dealing with a container (the thoracic cage) which is itself subject to a variety of osteoarticular restrictions. This container encloses essential organs (lungs, heart, etc.) which often give rise to symptoms similar to those of the container.

In this section on pathology, we shall mention some typical diagnostic mistakes made when working with the thorax. Some are obvious and straightforward, others less so and require significant knowledge and skill to detect. As mentioned repeatedly in our previous books, you should never hesitate to refer your patient to a specialist when you have reason to suspect malignancy or other serious disease. Sometimes the worst X-ray is more valuable than the best pair of hands.

Based on our clinical practice, we have compiled a list of characteristics of mechanical (osteoarticular and soft tissue) problems which help distinguish them from more physiological or psychological disorders. Obviously, there are exceptions in each case, and no injury is purely osteoarticular. Nevertheless, we have found this list to be useful, particularly when the characteristics are considered in combination.

Character of the Pain

- The quality of mechanical pain does not change rapidly. Mechanical pain is latent and can last a long time. Be wary of pain which is repetitive and changeable, particularly if it becomes more generalized.
- Mechanical pain increases with active movement but remains relatively localized during mobility tests.

Relationship between Pain and Activity

- Rest and immobilization of the painful part brings relief from mechanical pain.
- Nocturnal pain due to mechanical causes is rare, especially between midnight

and 3AM, but sometimes resumes after 4AM, in association with increased vagal activity. The mechanism for this commonly-observed phenomenon is unknown.

Related Signs and Symptoms

- In pain from mechanical causes the color of the skin, lips, and eyes is normal. There should be no fever or enlarged lymph nodes. If someone who you think has mechanical pain also has signs of an infection or respiratory problems, you should think very carefully about your diagnosis.
- Mechanical pain does not cause intense fatigue, sweating, or agitation, nor is it accompanied by anxiety. Pain associated with great anxiety is likely to reflect a more serious illness.
- Mechanical pain is relatively localized, usually affecting only one or two costal or vertebral segments.
- Mechanical pain may be aggravated by coughing, sneezing, or physical effort, sometimes making it difficult to tolerate. However, there is no lasting radiation into the thorax.
- Mechanical pain due to vertebral or costal restrictions is rare in young children.

A mechanical problem, compared to a visceral problem, is less likely to have significant or long-lasting effects on arterial pressure and pulse. For example, while a restriction of C5 may increase systolic pressure to 140 mm Hg, such an effect is likely to be transient. A kidney restriction can increase the pressure to 190 mm Hg, for a longer period.

It is also important to remember that pain due to visceral dysfunction seldom precedes joint pain; when it does, this can indicate a serious problem. For example, sore throat which follows cervical pain can be due to cervical dysfunction. On the other hand, a sore throat which precedes joint pain is cause for greater concern.

We must mention here that Pott's disease (kyphosis resulting from tubercular osteitis of the spine) is an absolute contraindication for manipulation. However, signs of this disease are usually obvious, and the disease itself is quite rare these days.

General Examination

We will discuss general clinical diagnosis in this section, and focus on osteopathic diagnosis in Chapter 5. When a patient consults a practitioner of manipulation for a thoracic problem, it typically involves perceived costovertebral pain. Of course, certain osteoarticular restrictions can produce dyspnea, side pain, intercostal neuralgia, precordial pain, or mediastinal pain. However, these symptoms may hide more serious illnesses where early diagnosis is crucial. Since we typically see these patients soon after symptoms first appear and before the disease has progressed very far, it is very important to reach the correct diagnosis, and make a prompt referral to a specialist if appropriate.

We were hesitant to include a section on medical diagnosis. This section is long, perhaps too cursory in some parts and overly detailed in others, and not an adequate substitute for a good grounding in internal medicine. We have generally avoided duplicating the efforts of standard texts as much as possible. Information from a book obviously cannot replace clinical experience. To be honest, we were more interested in writing the osteopathic sections in Chapter 5. Realistically, however, in our practice we treat patients with all types of pathologies. The question of which type is "our business" and which is not is often academic. Differential diagnosis is quite difficult and careless mistakes can easily pose danger for the patient. Some use this to support their claim that osteopathy should only be practiced by physicians. We feel that while medical diagnosis is difficult, it is not more so than manual practice. To the best of our ability, we should learn both. This section, therefore, summarizes relevant conventional medical approaches, together with insights and comments from our osteopathic perspective.

HISTORY AND PHYSICAL

In dealing with suspected thoracic pathologies, it is important to observe general (nonspecific) signs in addition to specific ones. The patient's attitude, complexion, etc. can provide important clues. For example, patients with thoracic problems often have a pronounced slouch, with the shoulders down and rotated anteriorly, and typically show or report some combination of the following: pale complexion, fatigue, rapid pulse, abnormal blood pressure, feverishness and shiver, agitation, profuse perspiration, weight loss.

The history should include a description of the pain (localization, onset, and intensity) and any respiratory difficulties. If there is a cough, you should obtain a complete description of it, i.e., its rhythm, quantity, quality, and whether it is productive or not. For example, with left ventricular insufficiency, the cough is nocturnal and exaggerated in the supine position.

During the examination, check carefully for abnormal respiratory noises such as crowing (laryngotracheal whistling noise), stridor (noisy respiration with snoring noise), and sibilance (whistling noise with respiratory murmur).

VISUAL OBSERVATION

Observe chest expansion, looking particularly for an imbalance of respiratory amplitude between the two hemithoraxes, which may reflect various problems. For example, mobility of a hemithorax can be inhibited by a hepatic problem (which affects the right side) or a costal restriction. In the latter case, inhibiting the rib in the direction of ease will usually lead to a restoration of normal mobility.

Edema localized at the base of the thorax is a sign of pleuritis, while edema in the upper thorax may reflect mediastinal vascular compression. Collateral superficial venous circulation which is unilateral in the clavicular regions indicates compression of the venolymphatic system by a tumor or mediastinal aneurysm.

PALPATION

Osteopaths are very good at palpation, but we tend to focus on a search for somatic dysfunctions. In the thorax (and elsewhere) this is not sufficient. Besides knowing if the problem is superficial versus deep, we must also discover if it is primarily muscular, nervous, mediastinal, or visceral.

Costovertebral mobility tests are instructive but cannot eliminate diagnoses of possible deeper pathologies. Consider a unilateral costovertebral restriction, detected at the level of the lowest costovertebral articulations. While this could indicate a simple musculoskeletal dysfunction, we also know that unilateral contraction of the paravertebral muscles at this level can result from pleural inflammation.

Direct palpation of the thorax can be very helpful in diagnosis. One such test in known in France as Rualt's sign. This involves placing both your hands on the patient's shoulders and asking him to inhale. A positive sign (palpably jerky or late expansion of one of the pulmonary apices) is associated with the early stage of tuberculosis. Friction rubs (rubbing between the two layers of the pleura when they are pathologically involved) provide another important piece of information.

Sometimes palpation reveals subcutaneous emphysema in the lateral cervicothoracic areas, a possible sign of pneumothorax. However, we have experienced only ten such cases in which all other examinations were negative. Interestingly, all of these cases involved restriction of the cervicothoracic junction. We had the impression that these restrictions sometimes cause subcutaneous emphysema following effort.

ISOLATED CERVICAL ADENOPATHIES

These are very visible signs for which the patient demands an explanation. Chronic lateral cervical swelling (especially in patients without any previous history of acute inflammatory swelling) could correspond to swollen lymph nodes, a congenital cyst, or a nervous or (very rarely) vascular tumor. Congenital cysts, the most frequent cause, are seen mostly in asymptomatic adolescents or young adults. Such cysts often appear as a single firm mass that fluctuates in size and yields slightly to mobilization. They are most frequent during growth phases, and are not painful.

With increasing frequency, we see young patients who complain of acute cervical pain without any history of unusual effort or trauma. Mobility tests are nearly impossible to carry out because the pain is so intense. Do not attempt to manipulate these patients! Palpation reveals numerous small nodes resulting from an infection, and the cervical pain resolves spontaneously within a few days. We must emphasize that articular pain of purely traumatic origin in children is very rare, apart from falls on the coccyx or "rolls" during gymnastics or other sports.

In adults, the presence of lateral cervical or supraclavicular swellings (called Troisier's node on the left) that slowly spread can correspond to a nodal localization of a malignant tumor. When the cervical nodes are involved, problems are usually found in the cervical fascia, mediastinum, or lungs; when the supraclavicular nodes are involved, problems are likely to be found within the abdomen. Lymphadenopathy of infectious origin is usually found in young adults, and the mass is firm rather than hard.

MUSCULAR ATROPHY

We occasionally see patients with partial or total muscular atrophy. Often this condition has been present for a long time but has been largely ignored. Viral infections (e.g., influenzas) can destroy parts of the peripheral nervous system. The patient may complain only of cervical pain or cervicobrachial neuralgia, and you will have to deduce the missing signs. Healing will take place either spontaneously or not at all. Each year we see about five cases of deltoid paralysis, varying in extent, following cases of influenza. Be sure to check the deep tendon reflexes of the deltoid, biceps, and triceps muscles and perform further evaluation as necessary. Tests of nervous system function will be discussed in Chapter 5.

Pulmonary System

VIBRATORY PALPATION

During palpation of the thorax, it is important to notice variation in vibrations on the chest surface, which can provide valuable information. Increased density of the pulmonary parenchyma increases the conductibility of vibration. Presence of liquid or gas between the parenchyma and chest wall reduces vocal vibrations. So do obstacles to bronchiolar ventilation, or loss of alveolar elasticity.

A common test for vocal vibration is tactile fremitus. Sit the patient down and ask him to say "toy boat" each time you touch him. (This test is easier to carry out on people with deep voices.) Place the palm of your hand over various regions of the lungs and compare the vibrations as the patient speaks. In most people, the slight vibration you feel will be more perceptible on the right anteriorly and in the right interscapular area.

Increased tactile fremitus is a sign of consolidation (solidification of lung tissue into a firm, dense mass), which may occur in pneumonia, pulmonary congestion, tuberculosis, or at the center of a pulmonary embolus. Decreased fremitus indicates an obstruction in the bronchial system, or that the lung is being pulled away from the chest wall, such as by a slight pleural lesion or emphysema. Pleural effusion can lead to impalpable local vibrations, as can pneumothorax or pachypleuritis (thickening of the pleura by highly vascular connective tissue, often seen in cases of chronic pleuritis). An effusion can also lead to consolidation higher up in the lung, with resulting increase in tactile fremitus.

PERCUSSION

This technique enables us to evaluate regional differences in sonority of the thorax and its contents, with comparison of the two sides. Sonority is affected by presence of intrathoracic viscera; e.g., the cardiac and hepatic regions have the dullest response. Percussion is performed with the patient seated and the back rounded to open the posterior intercostal spaces, or in the supine position for testing of the anterior chest. Lack of resonance on percussion can signify modification of parenchymal tissue, or presence of liquid between an organ and the chest wall.

Absolute dullness signifies:

- an area of significant pulmonary consolidation, pneumonia, or congestion;
- localized liquid effusion, pleuritis, pericardial effusion, subpleural edema, or splenopleuritis (congestion of the lung due to a streptococcal infection or tuberculosis, producing a resemblance to splenic tissue, without effusion but with edema).

Slight dullness signifies:

- an area of deep consolidation covered by normal parenchyma, as seen with pulmonary abscesses, congestion, pneumonia, or tumors;
- multiple centers of a disease distributed within healthy parenchyma, e.g., bronchopneumonia, tuberculosis, neoplasms;
- atelectasis (collapse of the pulmonary alveoli with loss of ventilation but continued blood circulation), or partial sclerosis.

Dullness of a specific area signifies:

- pleural effusion, if there is a well-defined upper limit which changes with position;
- pleuritis and thickening of the pleura, if there is dullness or slight dullness with poorly-defined upper limit which does not change with position.

Abnormal sonority signifies:

- emphysematous distension of the parenchyma, if bilateral;
- pneumothorax, if unilateral;
- pleuritis or hydropneumothorax if there is a slight tympanic noise above a zone which is abnormally dull ("Skodaic resonance").

The area of percussive dullness due to the heart occupies a roughly triangular zone limited by the right edge of the sternum. The superior border of the area of hepatic dullness runs from rib 5 on the right to around the fifth intercostal space on the left. This area contains a zone of absolute dullness, located at the medial part of the fourth and fifth intercostal spaces, in direct contact with the apex and convexity of the heart. Modification of these dull areas often accompanies abnormal visceral position due to significant parenchymal lesions, pleural retractions from scarring, or major effusions. You should be aware that:

Skodaic resonance is an area of hyperresonance above a pleural effusion. It is important to realize this and not make the mistake of thinking that the normal side is "dull."

Ellis' curve is the S-shaped curved line (revealed on percussion) reflecting the superior limit of dullness resulting from a pleural effusion.

Grocco's triangle is a triangular area of relative paravertebral dullness at the base of the thorax, on the opposite side from a pleural effusion.

AUSCULTATION

Auscultation means listening to sounds within the thorax, either directly or through a stethoscope.

Modifications of Breath Sounds

Vesicular (also known as alveolar) breath sounds are the normal sounds heard over the peripheral lungs fields. Diminished vesicular breath sounds are associated with decreased permeability to air of the pulmonary parenchyma, or with decreased amount of air entering the auscultated area, which occurs in cases of hyperemia, blood stasis, pulmonary edema, loss of alveolar elasticity, bronchial obstruction, parenchymatous destruction, paresis of the inhalatory muscles, or presence of liquid or gas between the lung and chest wall. No pathological process can cause vesicular breath sounds to be heard from areas from which they are not normally heard.

All other types of breathing sounds are called adventitious sounds. The most common adventitious sounds are wheezes and rales. Wheezes are continuous and usually signify bronchiolar disorders. Rales are interrupted and can be due to many different causes. One way to simulate the sound of rales is to rub hairs together close to your ear. Rales heard early in inhalation are usually due to obstructive pulmonary diseases such as bronchitis, asthma, and emphysema. Those occurring late in inhalation indicate pneumonia, congestive heart failure, or fibrotic processes.

Tubular (or tracheal) breath sounds, in a healthy subject, are heard over the trachea. Their audibility at the periphery of the lungs is considered pathological because this implies a solid connection between the peripheral area and the trachea. A soft, distant, veiled, exhalatory, or shrill tone indicates pleuritis. It indicates the upper limit of pleural effusion, where the pulmonary parenchyma comes back into contact with the chest wall. A "bell" sound is heard in certain cases of pneumothorax.

Pleural Rubs

These pathological noises result from friction between the two pleural layers when they are inflamed. The noise is similar to that made by rubbing dry paper or new, untreated leather. The sound is neither eliminated nor modified by coughing, and is heard at the same time as thoracic expansion. Pleural rubs occur at the beginning or end of a case of pleuritis, while the layers are able to maintain contact.

Voice Abnormalities

Any voice abnormality is cause for concern and careful evaluation. They can be caused by consolidation processes of the parenchyma, nodal compression, or injury to certain nerves. *Bronchophony* is a deep thoracic resonance of the voice, as clear in the periphery as it is over the trachea. Causes and implications of bronchophony are similar to those of tubular breath sounds. In *pectoriloquy,* auscultation of the chest allows you to hear actual speech, not merely sounds. This provides a sensitive means of detecting consolidations. Check for pectoriloquy by having the patient repeatedly whisper a phrase with many sibilants, such as "sixty-six, please," while you auscultate first over the trachea and then the periphery, listening for similar sounds. Another voice abnormality, *egophony,* is revealed by asking the patient to say "bee." During auscultation, you hear the long "a" sound (as in bay) plus a loud resonance of the voice, as if someone is speaking in the patient's chest. This is typically heard at the upper limit of a pleural effusion.

DYSPNEA

This term refers to difficult or abnormal breathing. *Tachypnea* is rapid and superficial respiration. It is often compensatory and will resolve spontaneously; however, if it lasts for a long time and is very rapid it may indicate serious problems such as pneumonia, pulmonary embolisms, pleuritis, and pneumothorax. All of these diseases, because of pain or compensation, diminish respiratory amplitude and accelerate respiratory rate. Problems of cardiac origin can also lead to tachypnea. *Bradypnea,* or slow respiration, indicates restricted intake and output of air, not functional insufficiency of the parenchyma.

Dyspnea of mechanical origin can also occur. We often see patients with shallow breathing. If due to costal or costovertebral restrictions, this almost always involves disturbed inhalation. By inhibiting the restriction, you can immediately enable the patient to recover normal amplitude. Sometimes, with slight pleural effusions, just holding the two ribs over the effusion together to avoid movement can relieve the pain.

COUGHING

Painful coughing occurs with laryngitis or tracheitis, and at the beginning stages of pleuritis and pleuritis, when coughing worsens the pain. Dry coughs generally occur at the beginning stages of acute pneumonias and similar pathologies, before the secretory phase. In cases of pericarditis and pleuritis, coughing is noticeably aggravated by changes of position.

Coughing fits may indicate mediastinal irritation or compression, tracheobronchitic adenopathies, or cardiac problems. Of course, they can also result from pertussis (whooping cough), a bacterial disease primarily affecting children.

Hemoptysis (coughing or spitting of blood) is in general a contraindication for manipulation. It occurs with tuberculosis, bronchiectasis, bronchial cancer, mitral stenosis, or upper digestive tract problems.

Costal or costovertebral restrictions can lead to a slight dry cough. A similar cough can occur after direct action thrusts to the thoracic spine (especially in the supine position), but is quite transient.

CHEST PAIN

This vague symptom has many possible origins, both non-respiratory and respiratory. The following lists are not intended to be comprehensive. Obviously, many of the causes are not susceptible to osteopathic manipulation, and call for appropriate referral.

Non-respiratory Origin

- Osteoarticular pain following direct or indirect trauma. This includes reflex pain from the cervical spine.
- Injury to peripheral nerves, especially the phrenic, vagus, or intercostal nerves. This can be accompanied by skin changes (sometimes painful) in the dermatome of the nerve in question, e.g., herpes zoster.
- Myositis (many causes).
- Osteitis (inflammatory, neoplastic, or infectious).
- Breast problems, including mastitis and mastodynia (neuralgic pain of the breast from various causes such as abscesses or malignancy).
- Rheumatic pain from, e.g., non-articular rheumatism of ankylosing spondylitis.
- Mediastinal problems such as tumors, Hodgkin's disease, or esophagitis. In the early stages, these may present only local discomfort.
- Gastric problems such as ulcers, gastritis, ptosis, hiatal hernia, gastroesophageal reflux, or aerophagia.
- Numerous disorders of the liver, gallbladder, appendix, colon, spleen, kidneys, ovaries, or other abdominal organs can also produce chest pain. Scapulohumeral pain sometimes results from urogenital disorders via the peritoneum. Similarly, scapular/thoracic pain can be provoked by culdoscopy or hysterosalpingograms.
- Precordial pain of psychological origin is usually localized very near the surface projection of the superficial cardiac plexus, at the level of the second and third intercostal spaces.

Respiratory Origin

The parietal pleura is very sensitive, and problems involving the pleura often produce chest pain. When upper back pain is due to pleural disorders, it is aggravated by coughing or deep inhalation. In acute serofibrinous pleuritis, pain is centered near the bottom of the chest and extends upward as far as the axillary region. In dry pleuritis (those with a fibrinous exudate, without the effusion of serum) the pain or twinge in the side is more limited and superficial, resembling intercostal neuralgia. The pleura is also a source of pain with spontaneous pneumothoraxes, which will be discussed later.

Problems with the parenchyma of organs usually do not produce pain directly, but via resultant irritation of the pleura. Pain from simple pneumonia is typically felt in the lateral midthorax, and is sudden and intense. When pain is low and on the right, it may signify appendicitis, cholecystitis, cholelithiasis, or even renal lithiasis. Localization of pain in many other areas can result from such problems as pneumonia, abscesses, tumors, or tuberculosis. As this is not an internal medicine text, the above list is far from exhaustive and mostly confined to situations we have encountered in our own practice.

Other Common Causes of Thoracic Pain

Our clinical experience has shown that upper back and chest pain can be due to relatively serious internal pathology. From the list above we have most often seen pleuritis, spontaneous pneumothorax, neoplasms, or tuberculosis. We have sometimes been the first to diagnose such diseases. You have a similar responsibility as a health care provider, and to emphasize this we will briefly describe some of these serious diseases which you are likely to encounter in your practice of osteopathy. Naturally, you will need to consult a specialized internal medicine text for further details.

In theory patients consult osteopaths because of joint problems, not for intrathoracic visceral conditions. However, symptoms during early stages of cardiac or respiratory diseases may be similar to those resulting from mechanical problems. We have seen patients with cancer or tuberculosis who consult us for such problems as upper or lower back pain, scapulohumeral periarthritis, or cervical pain. Early, correct diagnosis in such cases can literally be the difference between life and death. This is why you must be familiar with the signs of several serious thoracic pathologies. Having wonderful "hands" does not excuse you from missing important diagnoses. When a patient presents with chest pain, you have to decide whether you are dealing with coronary artery disease, an asymptomatic infarct, costochondral restriction, or precordial pain caused by anxiety. As another example, effort-induced pneumothorax can produce the same symptoms as a restriction of C7/T1.

In the next few pages we will briefly describe some serious thoracic diseases which we have encountered in our practice. Cardiovascular pathologies will be discussed in the following section. Even if the probability is small that you will come across these, we hope the confidence of being prepared to help your patients in unusual as well as routine cases will be sufficient incentive for you to learn this material.

SPONTANEOUS PNEUMOTHORAX

We have encountered ten cases of spontaneous pneumothorax. These patients consulted us for cervical or upper thoracic pain with anterior or posterior intercostal radiation. Interestingly, three cases involved people who had gone wind-surfing in strong winds. Mobility tests revealed muscular/ligamentous restrictions of the cervicothoracic junction but with some possibility of movement. The restrictions were more frequent on the left. Respiratory signs were slight or even nonexistent. Differential diagnosis will be discussed in Chapter 5.

This condition is often caused by a rupture in the pleura around an emphysematous subpleural bubble, or by a pulmonary breech resulting from a fractured rib which has perforated the pleura. Pleural or alveolar rupture may follow severe and rapid compression or elongation of the thoracic wall if the alveoli are distended and the glottis closed at the moment of impact. Sometimes, with forced movements of the arms and cervical spine, certain superior fibers of the pleura are stretched, causing small ruptures. These fibers usually belong to the cervicopleural system and become slightly fibrosed during palpation. We are certain that numerous minor cases of spontaneous pneumothorax evade detection and resolve themselves, while the patient is treated to diagnoses of cervical pain, cervicobrachial neuralgia, or scapulohumeral periarthritis of unknown origin.

In severe forms of spontaneous pneumothorax, signs include violent unilateral pain with lateral radiation (accompanied by dyspnea and dry coughing fits), silent hemithoracic respiration, sonority with percussion, abolition of vocal vibrations, amphoric breathing, and pectoriloquy (or more rarely, a metallic tinkling sound). Other, more obvious signs include sweating, cyanosis, tachycardia, tachypnea, and subcutaneous emphysema which, on palpation, feels like little bubbles of crepitant air under the skin.

In less severe forms there may be shallow thoracic respiration, cervical pain, and/or shoulder pain. The pain develops quickly and is often related to sustained activity or intense physical effort. In the fairly typical case we encountered most recently, the patient had spent two days wallpapering a ceiling. When the arms are in the air and the head leans backward, the pleura is significantly stretched. The next day he experienced pain in the left arm reaching to his fingertips. Physical examination revealed the following:

- left antalgic attitude of the cervical spine (left sidebending, slight right rotation, and superior left shoulder), with the left forearm pressed against the chest;
- in general listening he bent forward and to the left;
- it was impossible to bring the cervical spine into right sidebending and rotation;
- respiration was shallow but not rapid; deep inhalation was painful and nearly impossible;
- the left hand was edematous and faintly bluish in color;
- the systolic blood pressure on the left was 20mm Hg lower than on the right;
- C5, C6, C7 and T1 were restricted on the left;
- the Adson-Wright test was positive and there was miosis on the left;
- immediate relief was felt when the upper left hemithorax was compressed and lifted.

In our practice we do not usually see severe cases of pneumothorax, but rather minor, hard-to-diagnose cases without obvious symptoms. **Any manipulation in these cases is dangerous** because of the risk of extending the pneumothorax, which could lead to severe respiratory deficit; these patients must be sent to a hospital pulmonary department. In cases of minor pneumothorax (covering less than 20% of the pulmonary area), spontaneous closing is common, but these cases should still be kept under medical observation. After pneumothorax has completely resolved, we sometimes manipulate these patients.

GASTROESOPHAGEAL REFLUX

Here, we will discuss only the respiratory consequences of gastroesophageal reflux (GER). We estimate that at least 10% of the population will someday experience this disorder. The respiratory system is so commonly affected by GER that some practitioners believe that 60-80% of patients suffering from asthma and chronic bronchitis have this disorder, and it may even frequently be the cause of these diseases. There are some cases of "physiological" reflux, which last less than a minute and which are easily neutralized by salivary clearance. Atypical signs of GER, such as pharyngitis, morning hoarseness, otitis, or obstructive apneas in newborns, are complicated to diagnose because of the irregularity of reflux.

GER seems to act on the respiratory system in at least two different ways: directly through the acid reflux, or indirectly via the vagal system. The actual acid reflux that enters the lungs leads to bronchial hyperactivity. We believe that in cases of significant GER, the lower part of the esophagus is stimulated by acid reflux from the stomach. This, plus imbalance of tissues in this area, overstimulates the vagal afferent fibers, leading to a hypervagal state and possibly to a vicious cycle with continued gastric reflux, and so on.

In general, GER must persist for several weeks or months before causing noticeable respiratory problems. Be aware that the relationship between the lungs and gastroesophageal junction works both ways. Thus, any thoracic distension can cause decreased tonus of the lower esophageal sphincter and promote the development of GER.

Virtually any symptom of the pulmonary or ear/nose/throat systems can result from GER. For example, GER may irritate and lead to infection of the bronchi; if the infection is very severe, few people consider GER as the cause. We have been able to help many patients who had otherwise inexplicable disorders of the lungs or bronchi through successful reduction of their GER (see *Visceral Manipulation II*, pp. 55-56).

ESOPHAGEAL PAIN

There are chest pains, similar to angina pectoris, which can arise from problems of the esophagus. Approximately 20% of all patients with chest pain that is severe enough to justify cardiac catheterization have neither organic stenosis nor coronary spasms. In conventional medicine, more than 50% of such pain is attributed to the esophagus, particularly to GER. This differentiation cannot be clear-cut because of the relationship between the esophagus and heart. Not only do they share the same innervation, but there is an actual exchange of fibers between the esophagus and pericardium. With certain cardiac problems there are concurrent abnormalities of esophageal motility. Therefore, always be very careful with a patient who reports esophageal pain with swallowing. In osteopathy certain "cardiopathies" without well-documented organic disease can be explained by osteoarticular restrictions and injuries to the vagus nerve.

Consider GER in patients with recurrent pulmonary and related problems, including hiatal malfunctions. We can sometimes prevent development of esophagitis, which is well known for its carcinogenic risks.

LUNG CANCER

Lung cancer is the most common malignancy, especially in men between 50 and 70 years old. The ratio of male to female lung cancer patients is around 5 to 1. However, incidence of smoking by women has been rising steadily, and lung cancer, now the second most common cancer in women, will soon overtake breast cancer as the leading source of cancer mortality in women.

We have dealt with several cases of previously undiagnosed lung cancer in our clinic. Some patients consulted us only because of slight neck and upper back pain during the daytime that became severe at night. Always be wary of pain in the middle of the night!

With *primary tumors* the patient shows typical signs of a bronchial problem, but the nature of the cough is different. There may also be joint pain, fever, shivering, and wheezing. Hemoptysis is seen in less than 10% of cases. Sometimes there are no lung symptoms at all, and the patient will present with only prescalenic adenopathy, fatigue, anxiety, and the subjective feeling of having a serious illness.

More advanced cases, which we rarely deal with, involve acute weight loss, anorexia, nausea and vomiting. At this stage, pain becomes impossible to control. The voice becomes husky because of invasion of the recurrent laryngeal nerve (we may also see this sign at earlier stages, when the patient mentions a voice change).

Possible complications associated with lung cancer include pleuritis, dysphagia (due to esophageal invasion), diaphragmatic paralysis (due to phrenic invasion), Horner's syndrome (due to invasion of the cervical sympathetics), prescalenic or supraclavicular adenopathy, gynecomastia, peripheral neuropathies, atypical myopathies, purpura, and thrombocytopenia.

You should consider cancer in any patient over 40 years old with a lung problem which does not resolve in a reasonable period of time. Patients may report back and rib pain precipitated by a very slight effort. For example, one of our patients twisted his body trying to take a bag from the back seat of his car, and immediately felt excruciating intercostal pain. Mobility tests revealed a costal restriction, but our attention was drawn to the huskiness of the voice, presence of two large supraclavicular nodes, and tired aspect of the patient. Unfortunately, the radiographs we ordered confirmed our suspicions.

MEDIASTINAL TUMORS

Tumors of the mediastinum are usually asymptomatic, but may be accompanied by thoracic pain, dyspnea, and coughing. Neurogenic tumors are most common; malignant tumors are more frequent in children and almost always localized in the posterior mediastinum, along the anterior paravertebral groove.

Two-thirds of cases involve deep retrosternal pain, or upper back pain with costal radiation. The patient has no memory of any precipitant trauma or effort. Other telltale signs are diarrhea, hypertension, sweating, and flushing (repeated episodes of cutaneous vasodilation, particularly on the face). We must emphasize that **costovertebral pain in children is not normal.** This type of problem should encourage us to take chronic pain in children seriously and not reflexively come up with a diagnosis of normal "growing pains."

Superior vena cava syndrome is sometimes seen with mediastinal tumors in the upper thorax. This means that compression of this large vein results in edema and engorgement of the vessels of the face, neck, and upper extremities, along with facial cyanosis, sweating, nonproductive cough, and dyspnea. Sometimes a collateral superficial venous circulation appears in the upper thorax.

PRIMARY TUBERCULAR INFECTION

Primary tuberculosis occurs mostly in school age children. Even in developed countries, 75% of primary tubercular infections are never diagnosed. Patients usually come to see us because of pain of the lower neck or shoulders. Telltale signs are asthenia, anorexia, irregular bursts of fever, paleness, and fatigue. Long-lasting nose/throat or bronchial cold-like symptoms are also common. Advanced cases may involve prescalenic, retroclavicular, and axillary adenopathies, or erythema nodosum (multiple bilateral tender nodules, primarily on the anterior aspect of the lower extremities and, more rarely, on the upper extremities and face).

This disease is recrudescent, i.e., it may reappear a very long time after the first attack. We had one patient who consulted us for midback pain. According to the osteopathic literature, this problem is often associated with a duodenal ulcer. General listening, local listening, and manual thermal diagnosis all indicated a problem of the left pulmonary apex. The patient was surprised at this diagnosis and said, "I did have tuberculosis in the upper left lung, but that was 30 years ago." Nonetheless, a subsequent chest X-ray did show reactivation of the tubercular area. This case demonstrates the importance of performing a thorough exam even in cases of back pain where the visceral/somatic relationships may seem obvious.

DIAPHRAGMATIC DISPLACEMENT

The diaphragm may be displaced upward or downward depending on whether the origin of the problem is thoracic or abdominal. Note that the right hemidiaphragm is approximately 4cm higher than the left because of the presence of the liver. Upward displacement of one hemidiaphragm suggests an intra-abdominal mass, ascites, obesity, pregnancy, tumor, tumoral paralysis of the phrenic nerve, trauma, or infection. Often the mobility of the diaphragm is paradoxical, i.e., it goes up during inhalation and downward during exhalation. Downward displacement of one hemidiaphragm suggests pneumothorax or pleural effusion.

You may see one-sided spasms which reveal reduced mobility in one hemithorax. Such spasms usually result from problems of an attached organ, costal restriction, or more rarely, C4 or C5 restriction which has irritated the phrenic nerve.

With problems of the diaphragm, or the thorax in general, do not forget to check for hiatal hernias. They can have significant mechanical effects on the thorax, in part through their relationship with the diaphragm.

Cardiovascular Pathologies

With the cardiovascular system, as with the respiratory system, we make no pretense of describing every pathology you may encounter. We will mention certain disorders which show symptoms similar to those from an osteoarticular restriction, and important warning signs. Rather than advanced stages, we typically see early stages of cardiovascular diseases, when clinical signs are often misleading. We have had several dozen patients who consulted for pain in the cervical or thoracic spine but turned out to have real cardiac problems (particularly incipient coronary artery disease), even though all objective examinations and tests were initially negative!

Always consider cardiovascular problems in patients who report pain in the fourth and fifth left intercostal spaces, without significant intercostal restrictions. Such patients are often anxious, agitated, and have a vague sensation of being in danger. Surprisingly, we have found that most cardiac problems are accompanied by restrictions of C4-6 and

T4-6. Remember that with articular restrictions secondary to a visceral problem, a certain amount of mobility remains. This helps distinguish them from primary articular restrictions.

GENERAL SIGNS

It is essential that you learn as much as possible about reported pain. How did it first appear? Was it spontaneous and without apparent cause, or did it occur after a particular activity or effort? Did it occur after eating, during exposure to cold, during sleep, or during sexual activity? Localization of the pain is also important. Was it precordial, retrosternal, belt-like, or not localized? If it radiates, does it radiate to the arms, cervical spine, temporomandibular joints, lower jaw, diaphragmatic region, or abdomen? Finally, ask about the temporal nature of the pain. How long does it typically last? Is it relieved by rest, or by belching?

Another general sign for cardiovascular problems is dyspnea. This can be manifested as abnormal breathlessness out of proportion to the activity, or a nocturnal sense of oppression which prompts the patient to sleep on several pillows, sit up, or walk around.

We have seen several patients with coronary artery disease whose only symptoms were cervical or upper back pain. The most recent case only had slight, belt-like discomfort in the diaphragmatic region accompanied by a feeling of anxiety.

PALPATION AND PERCUSSION

Palpation of the heart in conventional medicine gives little useful information. One is only able to localize and evaluate the apical beat and its regularity, force, and extent. Normally, the apical beat is found on the midclavicular line between the fourth and fifth left intercostal spaces. It is due mainly to the withdrawal movement of the apex of the left ventricle.

Regarding percussion of the heart, please review the earlier discussion of pulmonary pathology. Importantly, the area of cardiac dullness should not extend past the right edge of the sternum. This roughly triangular area is delineated inferiorly by the horizontal line of hepatic dullness, and its left edge runs from the fifth left to the medial aspect of the second left intercostal space.

VASCULAR PROBLEMS

In Chapter 5 we shall discuss the Adson-Wright (Sotto-Hall) test, which has many diagnostic and therapeutic applications. Here we shall only mention some general signs of vascular pathologies.

Venous System

Warning signs during examination of the venous system include:

- distention, slow refilling of important vessels, swelling, cyanosis, or edematous infiltrations;
- a superficial collateral venous circulation, either thoracic or abdominal;
- the existence of a jugular venous pulse with systolic beats, or even hepatojugular reflux.

Note: cervical venous hum, a continuous sound like a spinning top heard over the internal jugular vein, is not considered pathological and should not be confused with heart murmurs.

Jugular venous pressure is not normally modified by 30-60 seconds' compression of the right hypochondrium. However, with right-sided weakness of the heart, this technique causes the venous beats to become stronger because abdominal pressure increases systemic venous return, the right ventricle cannot cope with the extra blood volume, and there is a resulting increase of pressure in the large veins. In cases of hepato-jugular reflux, pulsation of the internal jugular vein is observable when the hepatic region is compressed. This test is classically performed with the patient in the supine position with the torso lifted at 30 degrees, but can also be done using right subthoracic pressure in a seated patient.

Arterial System

You should be familiar with tests for hardening of the peripheral arteries. There are two signs associated with abnormal shock to the arterial wall. *Musset's sign* is nodding or shaking of the head in synchrony with cardiac movements in patients suffering from incompetence of the aortic valve, cardiac insufficiency (Alfred Musset, who described this sign, suffered from this condition), aneurysm of the aortic arch, or exophthalmic goiter. *Oliver's sign* is a pulsation of the aorta, distinctly felt through the cricoid cartilage in patients with aneurysm of the aortic arch. When looking for this sign, have the seated patient close his mouth and hyperextend his neck while you grasp the cricoid cartilage between thumb and finger.

Pulse Abnormalities

The arterial pulse is a source of much valuable information. You must always check pulse rate, looking for tachycardia or bradycardia, and also check for abnormalities of the rhythm or strength of the pulse. Pulses that are overly strong, feeble, or easily depressed are valuable warning signs. *Kussmaul's paradoxical pulse* is abnormal reduction of the pulse, associated with reduced systolic arterial pressure during inhalation. This may be a sign of mediastinitis, effusion, pericardial adhesion, or an obstruction to tracheal ventilation (e.g., croup, laryngeal stenosis). A *dicrotic pulse,* in which there are two successive systolic lifts for each arterial beat, is characteristic of aortic leaks and obstructive cardiomyopathies.

Takayasu's disease refers to obliteration of the major vessels coming from the aorta as a result of inflammatory panarteritis. Clinical signs include abolition of the pulse in both arms and the carotid arteries, intermittent claudication of the lower extremities, syncope, and problems of vision.

Simultaneous evaluation of the radial and femoral pulses gives information on arterial pressure of the lower extremities, which can be useful in osteopathy.

Hypotension

Aside from obvious traumatic causes such as acute hemorrhage, hypotension can result from anemia or acute infection. Fever often leads to a sharp drop in blood pressure. Low-grade fever coexisting with or following painful articular symptoms may represent acute rheumatic fever; in some cases there is no fever and only the pain is present.

It is very unusual for a child to report hip or knee pain without obvious traumatic cause; such cases must be taken seriously.

Always check your patients' blood pressure. In a patient with a history of ulcers, a systolic pressure drop of 20mm Hg or more may indicate a bleeding ulcer. We have seen three cases of acute upper back pain with hypotension which were really perforating ulcers. Be aware that when the bleeding begins the perceived pain may diminish.

COMMON CARDIAC DISORDERS

As usual, we will mention disorders with presenting symptoms that might suggest an osteoarticular problem, or those disorders which constitute a significant risk to the patient.

Precordial Pain

Precordial pain (i.e., pain perceived anterior to the heart) not involving actual cardiac injury can have several explanations. Precordial pain of *neurogenic origin* is seen in patients who complain of sudden, short pain not related to effort or other obvious cause. This pain, localized around the second, third, and fourth intercostal spaces, may be compared to the prick of a needle or thrust of a dagger, but without cervicobrachial radiation or anxiety. There may also be palpitations or arrhythmias. Such pain is often diagnosed as psychosomatic, but we caution you against jumping to this conclusion. Like many practitioners, we have initially suspected neurotic tendencies in patients who subsequently proved to have real cardiac problems. In women, precordial pain can be the first sign of malignancy or other problems of the breast.

Some cases of precordial pain are of *mechanical origin,* i.e., certain thoracic articular restrictions can produce symptoms similar to those of heart disease. A costochondral restriction, which is irritated by twenty-four thousand daily respiratory movements, can create inflammation of cartilages and ligaments and lead to pain that makes the patient believe he has a heart problem. Differential diagnosis for this situation will be described in Chapter 5. For now we will just mention that a true cardiac problem is almost always accompanied by a left cervical restriction. The mechanism for this relationship is unknown, but we may speculate that it is due to participation of the upper portions of the vertebropericardial ligament. We also believe that mechanical stimulation of the vagus nerve can cause coronary spasms, but have no definitive proof of this.

Precordial pain of *hiatal or gastric origin* often occurs consequent to a large meal or powerful emotion. In addition to radiation of pain to the heart region, one finds distension, stomach pain, and eructation. Differential diagnosis in these cases based on symptoms is difficult; local listening, in our experience, is of greater value. We believe that this type of chest pain is due to abnormal mechanical involvement of the cervicocardiac parts of the nervous system, vagus nerve, and the exchange of fibers between the hiatus and the pericardium. There is often anginal pain with hiatal hernias. Eructation may give temporary relief from pain in these cases, but can also give relief in some types of chest pain of cardiac origin.

Angina Pectoris and Coronary Artery Disease

Angina pectoris is due to a transitory insufficiency of oxygenated blood supply to the myocardium. The pain often begins during activity or effort, on going to bed, in the middle of the night, during sexual activity, or when getting up. It is usually constrictive, lasts only a few minutes, and is less localized than neurogenic precordial pain. It may be accompanied by severe anxiety and a sense of impending doom. A patient may report sensations of suffocation, something squeezing the heart, or a heavy weight on the chest. Sometimes the pain forces the patient to stop whatever he is doing and catch his breath. Overeating sometimes leads to crises of angina pectoris. Location of the pain varies: it is most commonly retrosternal, but may have a belt-like distribution. There is often radiation to the upper extremities, or even to the medial edge of the little finger. Sometimes there is pain in the jaws and throat without any thoracic symptoms.

In some cases of coronary artery disease (CAD) the patient exhibits few or no symptoms. We should be very careful with patients complaining of severe rib or back pain that affects breathing and comes without any apparent cause. Isolated jaw pain, not related to chewing activity, can also be a sign of angina pectoris or CAD instead of a bad bite. We have seen three patients undergoing treatment for TMJ syndrome in whom subsequent exams revealed CAD.

Myocardial Infarction

Myocardial infarction (MI), sometimes called heart attack, involves actual death of myocardial tissue due to obstruction of blood supply. The pain is more intense and long-lasting than that of angina, and sometimes becomes intolerable. It is described as heavy, squeezing, or crushing. Its onset is not always connected with effort or activity; patients usually cannot say what triggered it. When it occurs during activity, it is not alleviated by rest. Radiation of the pain is usually more clearly localized than that of angina; it may spread to the left arm, cervical spine, jaw, back, and abdomen (not below the umbilicus). Pain from MI often begins at night in association with a mild, transitory fever. The patient experiences weakness, dizziness, and nausea with or without vomiting. The crisis is accompanied by paleness, syncope, hypotension, and collapse.

At least 15-20% of myocardial infarctions are "silent" (without pain); since many such patients are never diagnosed, the proportion is probably even higher. The probability of silent MI increases with age. When these cases are symptomatic they start with dyspnea and (more rarely) confusion, and may also involve arrhythmia or a drop in blood pressure. The typical patient with MI is a man over 50 years of age who appears anxious, sometimes agitated, feels a need to belch or vomit, and twists his body. Other signs are weakness, paleness, sweating, cold extremities, and a rapid pulse in which the apical beat is difficult or impossible to find.

Pericarditis

This is inflammation of the pericardium, the membranous sac surrounding the heart muscle. Pain is similar to that of angina, including thoracic and retrosternal precordial pain, with possible radiation toward the cervical spine, neck, jaw, or left arm. Symptoms of pericarditis can also resemble those of pleural injury. We have seen three patients with pericarditis whose chief complaint was midback pain, radiating slightly toward the anterior thorax, which began suddenly without relation to effort or other apparent cause. We suspected an intrathoracic visceral problem in these cases because there was no articular restriction of the sternum.

Symptoms of advanced pericarditis include fever and pericardial rubs which sound like untreated leather. Unlike pleural friction rubs, which are synchronized with respiration, these are synchronized with the cardiac cycle. Of course, if there is simultaneous inflammation of pericardium and pleura, you may hear rubs synchronized with both cycles. In about 70% of pericarditis cases there is widespread cardiac dullness. The apical beat sometimes disappears, and in severe cases there may be a tamponade (acute compression of the heart by pericardial effusion). One sign of pericardial tamponade is a paradoxical pulse in which systolic blood pressure drops more than 10mm Hg during inhalation.

ARTERIAL DISORDERS

Aneurysm of the Aortic Arch

This is often discovered during routine examination. Symptoms include the diverse signs of mediastinal compression, deep and diffuse anginal pain, coughing, dysphonia (difficulty in producing speech sounds) due to compression of the recurrent nerve, and Horner's syndrome. Aneurysms are very difficult to diagnose; often the only initial signs are those of joint pain. We recently saw a patient with bilateral scapular pain not related to trauma or effort. We suspected a mediastinal problem, but CT scan revealed an aneurysm of the aortic arch. Unfortunately, this patient died during the operation. Even aneurysms of the abdominal aorta, which are theoretically palpable, are difficult to diagnose. We have seen four of these cases, in most of which the only obvious symptom was low back pain. One case required immediate surgery.

Narrowing of the Aorta

Narrowing (coarctation) of the aortic lumen can occur anywhere, but is most frequently seen above the origin of the left subclavian artery, near the insertion of the arterial ligament. A subductal coarctation (under the arterial canal) gives few symptoms, e.g., headache, cold extremities, or intermittent claudication. Sometimes on routine examination the patient is found to have a cardiac murmur or hypertension of the upper extremities only. In contrast, the lower extremities show lessening, delay, or absence of femoral pulsations, and low or absent arterial pressure. Palpation in an adult reveals dilated and pulsating collateral vessels in the anterior intercostal spaces, axillary fossae, or interscapular regions. A mid-systolic murmur is audible over the anterior part of the chest, back, and spinous processes.

Arteriosclerosis and Other Disorders

Arteriosclerosis is a degeneration of the muscular fibers of the arterial wall, with hardening and loss of elasticity, seen mostly in renal and muscular arteries. In patients with this problem one feels the sinuous aspect and classic pipe-like hardening of the radial, humeral, and temporal arteries. These signs are easily confused with signs of hypertension, which often occurs in the same patients.

Atherosclerosis is a form of arteriosclerosis characterized by lipidic deposits found on the intima of the vessel, followed by sclerosis and calcification of the elastic fibers. The violence of the ventricular contractions in these patients, and also the sharp intra-arterial loss of pressure which follows, is clearly demonstrated by the abnormal mobility of the superficial arteries, and by Musset's sign.

Arterial *hypotension* is revealed by instability of the pulse with a noticeable variation in radial pulse frequency, particularly when arising from a recumbent position.

Dissection of the vertebral artery, a less-common arterial disease, is of interest in manual therapy because it is perhaps the only one that can make cervical manipulation dangerous. This condition, which involves cleavage of the middle, circumferential or longitudinal tunic, results from degenerative lesions of the media with destruction of the elastic fibers. Mechanical pressures are high in the bend in the vertebral artery between C2 and the occiput, and vertebral arterial ruptures have been reported after manipulation or in subjects (e.g., painters) who worked for long periods with the arms in the air and head backward. Vertebral artery dissection presents few symptoms; these may include vertigo, headache, or slight loss of balance. Mobility tests do not show significant restrictions of the cervical spine. Never manipulate vertebrae that are not restricted; this may lead to serious problems. Also, do not manipulate the cervical spine in hyperextension; this can decrease blood flow to the cerebrum by about 30%.

Breast Disorders

We have never encountered a disease of the thymus, and therefore see no point in discussing this organ here. However, we would like to mention some problems of one other thoracic organ—the breast.

In our experience, breast disorders are almost invariably accompanied by cervical, thoracic, or costal restrictions, usually on the affected side. Be particularly wary when women come to see you for cervicothoracic pain localized around C4 and T4, with no history of trauma or other precipitating factor. Search carefully for nodules by palpation of the breasts, axillae, and clavicular fossae. We have had cases in which our suspicions about breast cancer were not borne out by medical examinations at the time, but in which the disease did unfortunately appear several months or years later.

With more advanced breast cancers, the patient often has sternochondral restrictions associated with cervicobrachial neuralgia on the affected side. These are the same restrictions found in a man with a cardiac disease. Treatment of the restrictions can sometimes alleviate some of the symptoms (e.g., back pain), but you must be aware that these restrictions are secondary. Severity of the restriction is usually correlated with severity of the underlying disorder.

Conclusion

It is admittedly uncommon that patients who consult us for osteoarticular problems subsequently are shown to have serious or life-threatening diseases. However, the possibility is always there, and we believe it is worth any effort to save a life. Be particularly on the look out for infarctions, which demand rapid diagnosis and treatment for the safety of the patient. In order of frequency, the serious diseases which we have encountered most often are:

- coronary artery disease (angina pectoris),
- spontaneous pneumothorax,
- pleuritis,
- primary tubercular infection,
- lung cancer,
- aneurysm.

Chapter Five: Manual and Differential Diagnosis

Table of Contents

CHAPTER FIVE

Manual and Differential Diagnosis

General Listening

General listening (or global listening) is a method of manually feeling tensions in the tissues. With practice, your hands will be drawn to the area where tensions are most significant. The tissues will "speak" to you, revealing the primary (or "least-secondary") restriction.

The patient should either be standing or seated, with the eyes closed to reduce outside influences. The body will move toward the side of the restriction with a sidebending movement accompanied, sometimes, by rotation. The restriction is found on the median of the angle formed by the sidebending of the vertebral column (see *Visceral Manipulation II*, pp. 8-11). Do not make the mistake of thinking that the rotation identifies the side of the restriction.

The mental attitude of the practitioner is crucial for effective use of listening techniques. You must be **passive** so as to receive only information coming from the patient's tissues. Simply receive the information at first, without trying to process it prematurely. You must have the conviction that your hand is going to "attract" the tissues, almost as if there was a magnetic force at work. The opposite is true of induction techniques, used to treat problems of motility. In the latter case, besides following the tissues, your hands are also following conscious instructions from your mind.

Our guidelines for general listening are as follows:

- The patient's body is always drawn to the side of the primary or most important restriction.
- The first movement you feel is always the right one. When a long time (more than a few seconds) passes before any movement is felt, there are three possibilities: the patient is free of restrictions (unlikely); the patient is not relaxing; or you are not sufficiently passive and therefore not listening effectively.

- Eliminate possible sources of interference with your listening, including any preconceived idea which causes you to unconsciously draw the patient into a certain position.
- When there is sidebending, the primary restriction usually involves the viscera; when there is simple forward or backward bending, the restriction is usually musculoskeletal. Rib restrictions are exceptions to this rule.
- Sidebending which finishes with rotation indicates a restriction in a more localized structure. For example, simple right sidebending which ends at the level of the liver usually indicates a general hepatic problem. If, at the end of the sidebending, there is a rotation to the left, this indicates problems of more specific structures, e.g., bile ducts or gallbladder.
- If the movement is extremely rapid or the tension is very light, the problem is likely to be primarily emotional.
- Be careful not to unwind the patient or perform myofascial release when you think you are listening. If the movement you feel seems too fast and has too great an amplitude, stop and then start again.

To perform general listening have the patient sit in front of you, legs hanging over the side of the table in order to eliminate information from the lower body. Place your dominant hand on the skull. Both your and the patient's eyes should be closed. The longitudinal axis of your hand should either be oriented along the anteroposterior axis of the skull (middle finger in the direction of the sagittal suture, palm on the occiput), or transversely oriented along the lambdoid suture. Restrictions in various areas will be revealed as follows:

Skull: A tendency of the hand on the skull to push inward is a sign of a sutural or intracranial problem. In four cases using this technique, we were the first to diagnose a tumor in patients who had previously had a negative work up complete with EEG and CT scan.

Cervical spine: The head goes into slight sidebending with slight rotation to the opposite side. With restrictions of the intertransverse muscles, or vertebral problems of the cervicothoracic junction, the head goes into backward bending and the end of the movement is concentrated on C7/T1. This is the common pattern following whiplash injuries.

Shoulder girdle and arms: The head undergoes large sidebending as if the parietal bone wanted to touch the shoulder on that side.

Pleuropulmonary system: We have considerable experience in this area. In general, the patient goes into forward bending and sidebending toward the side of the restriction. There is usually no rotation with superior pulmonary lesions, but rotation may occur with inferior lesions (which are less common). Rotation is often seen with pleural restrictions. To differentiate pleural from vertebral restrictions, simply inhibit the transverse process of the vertebra you think may be involved. If the problem is vertebral, this will cause the rotation to disappear. In order to confirm a pleural restriction, have the patient inhale deeply while sidebending and rotating toward the side of the suspected restriction (this positioning releases muscular tension). A pleural restriction is revealed by increased tension of the suspensory ligament felt during deep inhalation. You can also create an inhibition point at the apex of the pleural dome.

Heart: The head and upper back go into forward bending with slight left rotation. Differentiating cardiac problems from sternochondral restrictions is not easy. One method is to inhibit the suspected articulation during general listening. Disappearance of the movement you felt tends to confirm an articular problem. However, cardiac problems are sometimes accompanied by rib restrictions, and familiarity with the history and symptoms of the patient is therefore essential.

Breast: Problems of the breast and lung give similar results on general listening (i.e., forward bending and slight sidebending), but differentiating between the two is easy. If the breast is the problem, lifting it will eliminate the listening movement. It is rare that both breasts will simultaneously provoke a movement when listening, as one breast is always predominant. This is true for all paired organs.

Local Listening

After doing general listening it is necessary to do local listening to more precisely locate the restriction (see *Visceral Manipulation II,* pp. 11-12). This is done in a similar manner to general listening, but with the listening focused on a discrete area of the body. Local listening should not be restricted to the abdomen and thorax. One of the best ways to train yourself in local listening is to practice it on the upper extremities. The patient sits facing you, both elbows resting on the palms of your hands, the palms of his hands on your forearms (Illustration 5-1). Normally, you should feel the same resistance on both sides as you pull lightly on the elbows. When you release them, the elbows should both return to their original positions at the same speed. If there is a restriction of the shoulder or upper arm, the affected side will show relatively greater resistance to pulling and will

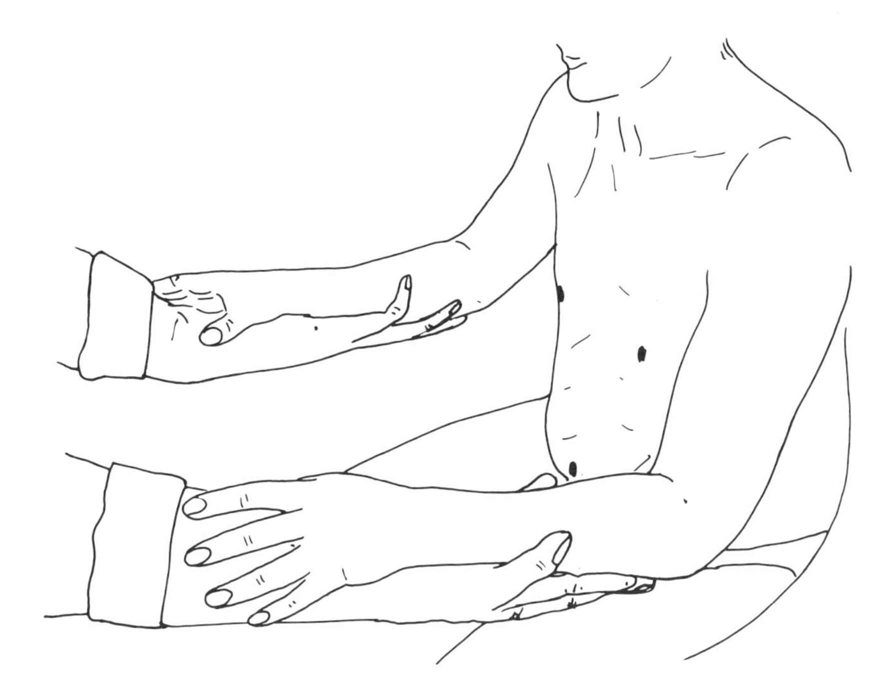

Illustration 5-1
Listening to the Upper Extremities in the Seated Position

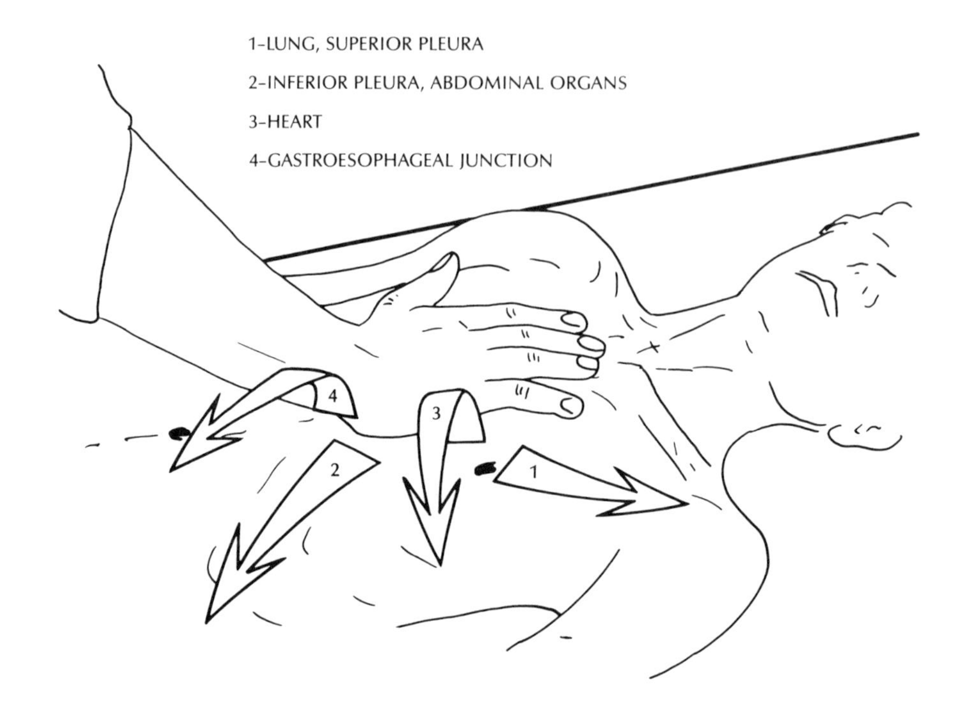

Illustration 5-2
Local Listening to the Thorax

return to the original position more quickly. By placing your hands in different places, you can focus your attention on specific areas. For example, placing your hands on the patient's elbows eliminates any information coming from the hands or wrists. If you want to include those areas, you need to place your hands more distally.

After doing general listening as described above, you will know which side the restriction is on, and its approximate location (thoracic or abdominopelvic). Local listening for the thorax is performed as follows.

Place your hand on the thorax of the supine patient, middle finger along the midline, and palm slightly above the xiphoid process (Illustration 5-2). We have experimented with local listening in the prone or lateral decubitus positions, but found this to be less effective. Let your hand passively slide to where the tissue restriction attracts it. Pay attention to the palm. It is always the movement of the palm which indicates the direction, and the restriction is located where the palm stops. When long distances are involved it may be necessary to carry out local listening in a step-by-step manner. For example, suppose that your palm is drawn toward the right as far as it can go but you still feel attraction in the same direction. Reposition your hand so that the heel of the palm is where the limit of movement was before, keeping the longitudinal axis of the hand parallel to the midline. Repeat this until there is no more movement and you will be over the restriction.

Guidelines for local listening are very similar to those for general listening:

- The patient's side, not yours, is the reference.

- Pure lateral sliding usually reflects a general visceral injury (e.g., of the right lung).
- Lateral sliding accompanied by either pronation or supination of the hand suggests a specific injury to a tubular structure (e.g., trachea, bronchi, blood vessels). We believe this is because of how a relatively localized restriction pulls the hand.
- A quick compressive movement frequently indicates an osteoarticular problem, specific pleuropulmonary restriction, or tumor. For example, with a sternochondral problem, the palm slides toward the articulation and stops abruptly against it.
- A rocking or see-saw movement which does not stop usually indicates involvement of a nervous plexus.

PLEUROPULMONARY SYSTEM

In local listening of the *lungs,* a restriction causes the palm to slide in the direction of the pulmonary apices. There is an initial sidebending and sliding of the palm toward the acromioclavicular joint, followed by a movement toward the middle of the clavicle. Whenever you are treating a patient with a documented pulmonary lesion, practice local listening to gain familiarity with these movements. To differentiate between lung and acromioclavicular restrictions, inhibit the latter joint. This is done by pushing the lateral end of the clavicle toward the acromion, releasing the ligamentous tensions. If movement on local listening is unchanged, the problem lies in the lungs.

With significant pleural injury, the cervicopleural attachments fibrose and contract, as we have often confirmed during dissections. In clinical practice, you must be able to differentiate between restrictions of the different pleural regions. Pleural problems generally give a stronger sense of pressure than costochondral or sternochondral restrictions.

With restrictions of the *superior pleura,* the palm is attracted toward the cervical spine and follows a line passing through the middle of the clavicle. The heel of the palm will stop at the level of the fourth or fifth costochondral joint. To confirm pleural injury, you can inhibit either the intertransverse muscles of the lower cervical vertebrae, or the cervicopleural attachment system, by using your thumb to push the first rib (located posterior to the middle of the clavicle) posteromedially. Another technique is to ask the patient to hold his breath in the middle of exhalation, which releases pleural tension. On the other hand, if you want to demonstrate pleural participation, ask the patient to inhale deeply in order to increase this tension.

With restrictions of the *middle pleura,* the hand moves very slightly toward the midthorax, or not at all. On local listening you have the impression that the hand is plastered against the thorax very quickly, as if attracted by a magnet. This movement is rather subtle and you will need some experience to feel it reliably.

With restriction of the *inferior pleura,* the hand moves posterolaterally toward ribs 8 and 9, and the palm stops at the level of the diaphragm. Local listening of the inferior pleura can be confused with that of the liver, stomach, colonic flexures, kidneys, or diaphragmatic hiatus. When this happens, inhibit the organ closest to the zone of pleural listening. You can also press an inhibition point located in the eleventh posterior intercostal space (where you can reach the pleura directly), ask the patient to hold his breath in the middle of exhalation, or inhibit the suspensory system. If the pleura is involved, any of these techniques will stop the movement.

Local listening of the *bronchi* is focused on the main bronchi, close to their point of intersection. With a restriction, the hand slides superiorly until the fingers are near the sternal angle, and the palm then moves outward from the midline. For the left bronchus, the hand and the midline form an angle of about 60 degrees to the left; for the right bronchus, the hand forms a 30 degree angle to the right. For the small bronchi, the hand presses against the thorax in a manner similar to that for costochondral restrictions, except with more pressure.

MEDIASTINUM

The mediastinum contains numerous arterial, venous, lymphatic, and digestive passageways. Local listening can only localize restrictions to this area, without being more precise. With a restriction, the hand moves superiorly, slightly compressing the sternum. This listening is very difficult to interpret because the mediastinum has so many components. In patients with sequelae of tuberculosis, particularly those with pleuromediastinal retractions, we also felt either pronation or supination of the hand, depending on the side of the restriction. In patients with Hodgkin's disease, we have noted that the hand flattens and is pulled straight posteriorly without rotation. However, our experience with this condition is limited.

CARDIAC SYSTEM

In patients with heart disease, local listening is fairly clear and easy to interpret: the hand moves slightly to the left while supinating. The larger the amplitude of the supination, the more serious the structural injury. Simple lateral sliding often indicates a slight functional problem.

By practicing with patients having documented coronary artery disease, we have learned that local listening may indicate which artery is affected. For the left coronary artery (or its branches, the anterior interventricular and circumflex arteries), the hand makes an angle of about 30 degrees with the midline on the left. The upper part of the hand is thus strongly attracted toward the second left sternochondral joint (see Illustration 2-20). For the right coronary artery, the hand moves to the right of the midline, forming a 40 degree angle having its apex at the second right sternochondral joint. With severe coronary artery disease the hand does not glide but is attracted straight posteriorly, as with a problem of the mediastinum. Always take advantage of the opportunity to train your hands by palpating a patient who has a history of infarct or coronary artery disease. Even if the lesions are old, the tissues never forget. Manual thermal diagnosis is also helpful in this kind of diagnosis.

Our experience with the *pericardium* is limited to about ten cases. Local listening here seems to be fairly precise. The only accessible part of the pericardium, i.e., without interposition of the pleura, is shaped like a small triangle. The summit is at the level of the fourth left sternochondral junction, the base at the level of costal cartilages 6 and 7, the right side at the left edge of the sternum, and the left side at the left costomediastinal recess. With local listening of pericardial problems, the palm is first attracted to this triangle, followed by a sensation that the apex of the triangle is trying to stretch up toward the superior thorax, while the base remains immobile. We believe this phenomenon is due to the cervicopericardial ligaments.

We have seen many cases of precordial pain related to the superficial *cardiac plexus*. This plexus has an important relationship with emotional tensions. On local listening the hand slides in sidebending toward the second and third sternochondral joints and does not move any farther. The palm is aligned inferiorly and to the left. In contrast to other local listening, at this point the hand continues to move in a clockwise or counterclockwise direction, or rocks back and forth, each time coming back to its original position. The frequency of movement is highly variable, probably averaging around twenty oscillations per minute. Sometimes one has the impression of feeling the cardiac plexus above the aortic arch before it distributes into the heart. More rarely, on local listening the hand flattens against the fourth and fifth intercostal spaces. We believe that this is due to dysfunctions of the intracardiac nervous system (nodes, bundle branches, etc.)

Finally, we should mention that we have often found problems of the gastro-esophageal junction associated with disorders of the heart or lungs, perhaps because of their shared vagal innervation. With restrictions of this junction, the palm is pulled to an area just below the xiphoid process, slightly to the left, and posteriorly.

Vascular Problems of the Thoracic Inlet

We have found that almost all neurovascular problems of the thorax are essentially vascular and localized at the thoracic inlet, a zone of natural compression where the large vessels are particularly vulnerable. On Adson-Wright testing (see below), we have noted positive results in approximately 20% of our patients. Although such a high

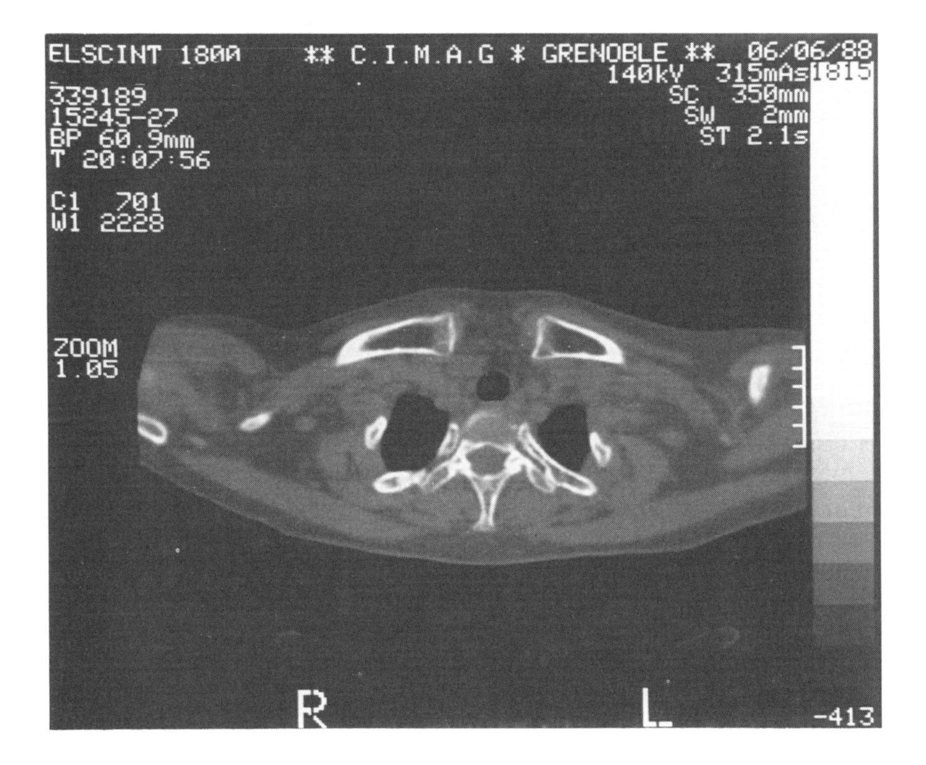

Illustration 5-3
CT Scan of the Thorax at T1 of Patient in Supine Position with Arms at the Sides

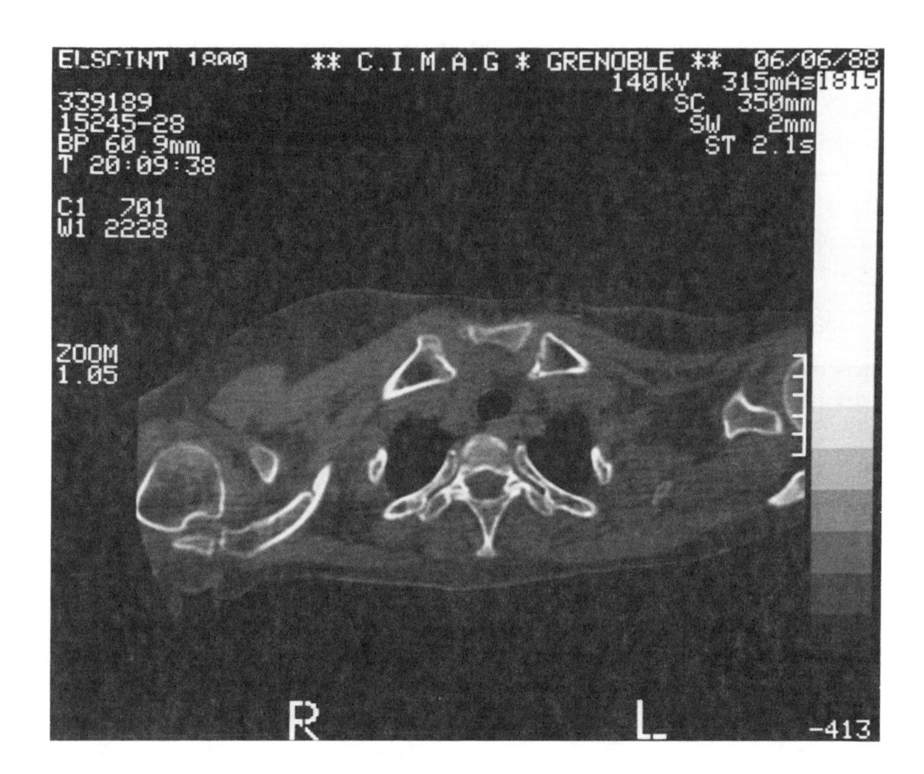

Illustration 5-4
CT Scan of the Thorax at T1 of Patient with Right Arm in Adson-Wright position

percentage is obviously cause for skepticism, there can be no doubt about the absence or presence of a pulse. Results of follow-up Doppler examinations in these cases did not always show vascular compression, but this could easily be due to the fact that Adson-Wright tests were incorrectly performed by the Doppler technician. For example, the test was often carried out in the supine position (which eliminates an important component of the soft tissue pressure), or the abduction and/or external rotation movement was omitted.

In *Visceral Manipulation II* we discussed experiments utilizing the Doppler effect and showing that a slight fascial release in the abdomen can have an immediate effect on blood flow through the subclavian artery. On the other hand, if the Doppler, which is essentially an arterial examination, shows no abnormality when a patient seems to have all the vascular symptoms of inlet compression, one could consider the possibility that some other vascular element is involved. Therefore, we used the CT scan to document what happens at the inlet during certain movements (Illustrations 5-3 and 5-4).

To begin with, we asked whether vascular compression is normally present in patients without functional problems of the inlet. We chose two subjects with a negative Adson-Wright and performed Doppler tests first in the supine position with arms along the body, then with an arm abducted and externally rotated, and finally with an arm in that position and the head rotated to the opposite side. We wanted to measure the diameter of the thoracic inlet and the length of the clavicle from the superior edge of the scapula to the transverse process of C7. These measurements were very difficult to obtain. However, after many trials we were able to document a narrowing of the thoracic inlet during the Adson-Wright movement. Several views showed clear compression of the subclavian vein and artery caused by backward movement of the clavicle.

Thus, as we suspected, the thoracic inlet is an area where vessels are **naturally compressed** in certain positions. For this reason, even slight degrees of myofascial tension may create vascular problems. We also confirmed our suspicion that the subclavian vein is typically the first vessel to be affected by such compression, and were able to explain numerous symptoms, similar to those of subclavian artery compression, in patients with negative Adson-Wright results. Compression of the subclavian vein is difficult to document by non-invasive tests.

ADSON-WRIGHT TEST

This test (also known as the Sotto-Hall test) was discussed extensively in our previous books. It consists of checking the radial pulse during a movement which brings the arm into abduction and external rotation while the head is either rotated to the opposite side or sidebent to the same side. The test is said to be positive if the radial pulse is reduced or eliminated. A positive result is obtained with all osteoarticular, visceral, and myofascial problems of the thoracic inlet. The test should be performed in the seated position so that the tissues are situated and functioning normally. The test should be followed by use of precise inhibition or aggravation techniques, which give information on why the test was positive (thus the phrase "completed Adson-Wright test").

Inhibition techniques consist of inhibiting tensions in the tissues by gentle pressure. Usually performed with a thumb or single finger, this is accomplished by pushing lightly in the direction you observed the tissue to move during listening. This pressure should stop, or inhibit, the direct or reflex tension in the tissues which causes the vascular problem. If inhibition restores the pulse during an Adson-Wright, the inhibited structure is likely to be the cause of the problem.

In contrast, *aggravation techniques* consist of exaggerating tension in the tissues by digital pressure, thus increasing the effects of the restriction. If the restriction is relatively slight, it may require aggravation before giving a positive Adson-Wright. In general, aggravation tends to emphasize and clarify effects of a problem in a particular structure. For example, supposed you obtain a positive Adson-Wright in a case where general and local listening, plus palpation, indicate a problem of the inferior insertion of the anterior scalene muscle on the scalene tubercle. The inhibition technique consists of placing the thumb on the inferior part of the muscle and pushing it slowly toward the tubercle, which moves the inferior fibers closer to their costal insertions. The aggravation technique is performed by pushing the first rib downward or stretching the muscle fibers upward, in order to increase tension. To use an aggravation technique in this case, release the external rotation of the arm until you come to the point where the radial pulse returns. Leave the arm in this position and, with the thumb of the other hand, exaggerate the tension of the anterior scalene by pushing the first rib downward. If the pulse again disappears, you have found the restriction. You will then have to follow up with differential diagnosis of the other soft tissues in this area, as they are all interconnected. We will explain how to do this later.

With a positive Adson-Wright, you will find that systolic arterial pressure of the injured side is often 10-20mm Hg lower than that of the other side. When this discrepancy is caused by a structural problem, osteopathic treatment will usually eliminate it in one session.

Osteoarticular Causes of a Positive Test

Osteoarticular causes of a positive Adson-Wright usually involve restrictions of the joints listed below. Other less common causes include clavicular osseous callus, enlarged transverse process of C6 or C7, or an overly oblique rib 1.

To find out if the *C7/T1 joint* is the cause of a positive Adson-Wright, create an inhibition point with the lower part of your thumb on the transverse process of C7 and the tip on the spinous process. The thumb presses gently toward the side opposite to the arm tested.

To evaluate the *first costovertebral joint*, create an inhibition of rib 1 by pushing its posterior portion anteromedially against T1. Aggravation is accomplished by irritating the stellate ganglion, i.e., compressing or squeezing it against the anterior surface of the transverse processes of C7 and T1.

Restrictions of the *sternoclavicular and first sternochondral joints* almost always occur together. After obtaining a positive Adson-Wright, you can use aggravation technique to check for this possible cause. Slowly release the external rotation of the arm until the pulse returns. Then, with the thumb of the other hand, exert posterior pressure on these two joints. If the pulse disappears again, the problem lies in these joints. Alternatively, you can use inhibition. Place the thumb against the inferior edge of the medial clavicle and press superomedially. If the positive Adson-Wright is due to a restriction here, the pulse will return. A third technique consists of pushing the sternoclavicular joint on one side to inhibit its counterpart on the other side and restore the radial pulse. This utilizes the interclavicular ligament to produce the inhibition.

Suppose you want to determine if a restriction of the third sternochondral joint is the cause of a positive Adson-Wright. Decrease the amount of external rotation just until the pulse returns. Then carry out an aggravation technique by compressing the third costochondral with a finger of your free hand. The force should be directed posteriorly and slightly laterally. If the cause lies in this joint, the pulse will immediately disappear. This test can also be carried out with inhibition by laterally compressing the sternal part of the third sternochondral in order to make the rib and sternum move together. Another inhibition method is to push rib 3 medially and slightly anteriorly.

Pure restrictions of the *lower cervical vertebrae* which lead to a positive Adson-Wright are not common. Cervical restrictions which affect the thoracic inlet are usually associated with problems of the middle cervical aponeurosis or pleura. To check for lower cervical restrictions, inhibit the intertransverse muscles and repeat the Adson-Wright test. The aggravation technique is more specific. Sidebend the patient's head slightly toward the side of the suspected vertebra. Then, pushing on the top of the head, focus the force on the specific interapophyseal joint. If your suspicion is correct, the pulse will disappear. This technique is useful in whiplash cases where the patient presents with vascular symptoms.

Myofascial Causes

As one looks at a sagittal view of the thoracic inlet, it is obvious that any spasm, adhesion, or fibrosis of the *subclavius muscle* contributes to compression of the inlet by bringing the clavicle closer to rib 1. This muscle can be injured by trauma to the thorax, but there is another important precipitating factor. Much of its innervation comes from the phrenic nerve which also contributes to abdominal, peritoneal, and thoracic visceral innervation. We believe that visceral irritations, because of reflex activity, often cause spasm of this muscle. This could explain the immediate results obtained after very gentle visceral manipulation, and also the inconsistency of these results. Because of the narrowness and high density of the inlet, which leaves little room for compensation, a simple muscular spasm is enough to compress it. If you suspect that the subclavius is the source of a positive Adson-Wright, compress the clavicle inferiorly and slightly medially to release the fibers. There is a more specific technique which is harder to carry out. Place your thumb in the supraclavicular fossa against the clavicle and the index finger of the same hand between rib 1 and the medial clavicle. In this position you can lightly pinch the subclavius muscle and thereby inhibit it.

Certain contractions of the *large muscles* which insert into the clavicle, particularly the scalenes and sternocleidomastoid, can also cause a positive Adson-Wright by decreasing the space between the clavicle and rib 1, or (e.g., in torticollis) between the clavicle and cervical spine. Such problems (except for congenital torticollis) are transitory and do not require treatment.

Fascial as well as muscular restrictions can cause compression of the thoracic inlet. You need to know how to use the completed Adson-Wright to determine exactly which tissues are involved. When the *middle cervical aponeurosis* is the cause, the Adson-Wright will be positive when the head is sidebent and rotated to the side opposite the arm being tested. There is a general test that can verify the involvement of this aponeurosis. The head is brought back to a neutral position or the arm lifted superomedially. This brings the clavicle and cervical spine close together and restores the pulse if the problem is in this aponeurosis. This technique will also bring back the pulse when the problem is in the suspensory ligament of the pleura. To make the test more specific, inhibit the aponeurosis by placing the thumb slightly above the scalene tubercle and delicately lifting it superomedially. With practice, you can create inhibition simply using the weight of your thumb.

The *suspensory ligament of the pleura* frequently causes problems of the thoracic inlet. Differential diagnosis can be done with the patient either passive or active. The passive method is to inhibit the pleural dome, which is located posterior to the anterior part of rib 1. This method makes it difficult to differentiate the pleura from the middle cervical aponeurosis. The active method, which is more specific, utilizes respiration. After obtaining a positive Adson-Wright, release the external rotation of the arm until the pulse just reappears. At that moment ask the patient to breathe in deeply. If the pleura is involved, the pulse disappears again because of the tension created by the suspensory ligament, which restricts the inlet.

Causes of a positive Adson-Wright related to the *pericardium and costomediastinal recesses* are difficult to differentiate. The patient sits in the Adson-Wright position, his back resting against your chest. Your free hand pushes the body of the sternum superiorly and slightly posteriorly. This releases all the components of the inlet and lightens the load of the soft tissues, as if the patient were weightless, and causes the pulse to return. Even if you find a restriction here, you must perform other tests to make sure that the problem is not located higher or lower.

Our experience indicates that inhibition of the *costodiaphragmatic recess* is not useful because this affects many other organs related to the diaphragm; i.e., inhibitory pressure on this recess will also inhibit the liver, right kidney, hepatic flexure of the colon, etc.

When dealing with thoracic inlet problems, be aware of the many abdominopelvic visceral restrictions discussed in *Visceral Manipulation* and *Visceral Manipulation II*, and their possible implications. In osteopathy, no part of the body is viewed as discrete or isolated. Each organ, muscle, tendon, bone, or joint is affected by every other tissue. Thinking that only problems of nearby structures can affect blood flow through the thoracic inlet is analogous to thinking that only disc herniation can cause sciatica.

Visceral Causes

In practice, we use the same inhibition and aggravation techniques for both the *lungs and pleura.* With severe pulmonary problems the following test for the fissures also tests for pleural restrictions via the ribs. The following description for the right horizontal fissure can be easily generalized to the others. The patient sits in the Adson-Wright position, his back against your chest. With your free hand compress the lateral aspect of ribs 5 and 6 inferomedially, going from the lateral edge of the scapula toward the fourth sternochondral joint. This releases the tension in the fissure and should restore the radial pulse. For the right oblique fissure, use ribs 7 and 8. Problems of the right fissures almost always cause a positive Adson-Wright on the right.

Problems of the *heart* cannot be differentiated from those of the pericardium and are difficult to separate from those of the pleura. There is an inhibition test for the upper part of the heart, but it is not precise. Place the palm of your hand on the second left sternochondral joint, with your fingers over the sternum directed toward the second right sternochondral, and pushing slightly posterior. The radial pulse should come back and will often speed up, this being one of the few techniques which cause cardiac acceleration. We are unsure that the effect here is restricted to the heart, since this technique utilizes the cardiac plexus.

The *gastroesophageal junction* should be kept in mind as a possible cause of intrathoracic problems. Diagnostic techniques are carried out while facing the diaphragmatic hiatus, with subcostal pressure applied just inferior to the seventh left sternochondral junction. First, the patient leans forward so that your thumb can be placed sufficiently posterior. The thumb then pushes the tissues which face the hiatus inferolaterally for inhibition, posterosuperiorly for aggravation. Do not confuse this technique with that for the celiac plexus, which is much more superficial.

Other Causes

There are many additional problems, besides those mentioned above, which can produce a positive Adson-Wright. Most involve the vascular system. In clinical practice, we have found an old cardiologists' maxim regarding vascular problems of the hand to be useful: white hand—arterial problem; blue hand—venous problem; painful hand—neurological problem.

Raynaud's disease is characterized by paroxysmal circulatory problems which lead to ischemia of the hands. The patient is particularly susceptible to cold, but episodes can occur during the summer as well. During ischemic attacks the fingers (usually not the thumb) are very painful and feel "dead." The underlying cause is poorly understood, but may involve the cervical sympathetic nerves. This disease should not be confused with Raynaud's phenomenon, which is always associated with other illnesses and is usually unilateral. Raynaud's disease gives a positive Adson-Wright but is usually bilateral, an unusual finding in problems due to increased tissue tension at the thoracic inlet. In fact, the pulse on the side opposite that of a positive Adson-Wright is generally stronger than normal. A bilateral Adson-Wright is frequently related to Raynaud's disease or other disorder of the sympathetic nervous system. For this reason, in such cases it is advisable to test the stellate ganglion. Place a thumb or finger very lightly against the transverse process of C7 just above rib 1. Gently press it toward the anterior part of the transverse process to inhibit the ganglion; to stimulate the ganglion, press harder.

Takayasu's disease, also called the pulseless disease, is a rare disorder of young women characterized by obliteration of the large vessels coming from the aortic arch, notably the subclavian. It is essentially due to an inflammatory adventitious lesion secondary to thrombosis. Common symptoms are abolition of the pulse in both arms and carotid arteries, intermittent claudication of the lower extremities, fainting, and problems with vision. There may also be anorexia, weight loss, fever, or night sweats.

We have noticed a positive Adson-Wright with several patients in with an *abnormal position of the radial artery.* In such cases, the radial pulse is located much deeper, sometimes more laterally or even on the dorsal aspect of the wrist. While performing the Adson-Wright be careful to always remain in contact with the artery, since the movement of the arm during the test can displace your pressure.

Adenopathy, which is an inflammatory reaction of the lymph nodes, can eliminate the radial pulse by compressing the subclavian or axillary artery, and perhaps via irritation of the nervous system.

Another possible cause of positive Adson-Wright is a disorder of the *subclavian, axillary, or brachial arteries.* The subclavian pulse can be felt (sometimes with great difficulty) posterolaterally to the scalene tubercle at approximately 1.5cm from the midclavicle. The axillary pulse is found between the clavicle and pectoralis minor muscle, near the coracoid process, outside the coracobrachial groove, or even within the axillary fossa. The brachial pulse is felt in the fold of the elbow, near the insertion of the biceps. If you suspect an injury to one of these vessels, refer the patient to a vascular specialist. A Doppler test is not an invasive procedure, and can reveal a vascular injury (thrombus, atheroma) requiring urgent treatment.

We have seen *thyroid* goiters large enough to come into contact with the supraclavicular fossa. Our most recent case was a young woman with a positive Adson-Wright on the right which was normalized by slight lifting of the right part of the thyroid. The only symptoms of a thyroid problem were hypotension, hyperthermia, and hyperreflexia. Confusingly, the symptoms of hyperthyroidism sometimes resemble those of hypothyroidism, and vary in relation with hormonal activity.

Mediastinal tumors can compress the large arteries, but typically produce other signs besides positive Adson-Wright, e.g., respiratory or retromediastinal symptoms, hypertension, and flushing (repeated episodes of cutaneous vasodilation, particularly of the face and upper thorax).

CLINICAL SIGNS OF VASCULAR COMPRESSION

Vascular compression of the thoracic inlet occurs only in certain positions: head leaning backward, arms in the air, one or two hands behind the head, or lateral decubitus position. It is almost never seen in a relaxed person in a neutral position. For this reason, the symptoms are labile and may improve or disappear with a change of position. They are probably the most pronounced upon awakening in the morning; often the subject has been sleeping in one of the positions mentioned above, e.g., one hand behind the head in lateral decubitus position. Try to pinpoint problems that are worst on waking up and improve as the day goes on. With such patients, test the radial pulse in lateral decubitus position by pushing the superior shoulder downward, which increases clavicular compression.

Subclavian Steal Syndrome

This is an interesting syndrome that develops when the subclavian artery becomes occluded and the major cranial vessels remain patent. In order to supply the arm, a reversal of blood flow takes place in the vertebral artery on the side of the occlusion. The patient shows typical symptoms of vertebrobasilar insufficiency: vertigo, nausea, loss of vision, double vision, or, in severe cases, loss of consciousness. Symptoms tend to be exacerbated by exercise of the affected arm, because the increased circulatory requirements of the arm "steal" more blood from the posterior part of the brain. Furthermore, exercise of the arm causes local pain because the circulation is still inadequate. Occlusion of the subclavian artery is almost always atheromatous.

Imagine a patient who suffers from compression of the subclavian artery in the thoracic inlet due to sleeping position. He may exhibit symptoms upon arising in the morning which resemble those of subclavian steal syndrome. The difference is that the decrease in the useful diameter of the artery is due to external compression rather than internal occlusion. Likewise, as circulation via the basilar arteries is also affected, symptoms may resemble those of actual injury to these vessels.

Local Symptoms

Local symptoms of vascular compression at the inlet are mostly due to arterial compression. The most common is a sensation of numbness (or pins and needles) of the fingers and arm. The fingers become white but are rarely swollen. Less commonly, there may be muscular problems. These symptoms are not permanent and the numbness should cease once the patient assumes a "decompression" position for the inlet. Usually this involves rotating the head toward the affected side while placing a hand on the opposite shoulder. If this does not alleviate the symptoms, a thorough vascular examination is necessary.

As mentioned earlier, the subclavian veins are usually the first vessels to be affected by a narrowing of the inlet. Signs of subclavian vein compression are swollen, bluish fingers, pins and needles sensation, sticky hand, pitting edema of the hand and arm, and, more rarely, lateral cervical and ipsilateral supraclavicular edema. We have seen three patients suffering from such compression in whom the arm was so swollen and heavy that it had to be held in a sling, but generally the problem is less severe. Be sure to rule out lymphedema due to tumor in these severe cases.

General Symptoms

There are many non-specific problems that can arise due to vascular compression of the inlet. One of the most common is *headache.* This is mostly posterior initially but may spread as far as the frontal region. Subclavian problems often affect the vertebrobasilar artery, as discussed above. In general, we like to see patients with headaches which begin posteriorly, since these are often due to mechanical problems and respond well to manipulation.

Vertigo associated with compression of the inlet is often of the type triggered by changes of position, particularly from standing to lying down. This type never occurs when the patient is lying down, or when he rises to his feet. This vertigo is transient but makes the patient very anxious because there is a strong feeling of "fading out." Be very careful with patients whose vertigo is not positional.

Vertigo related to inlet compression also often begins during activity with the arms in the air and the head bent back; in this position blood supply to the vertebrobasilar artery is reduced due to compression of the subclavian artery, as well as of the vertebral artery as it passes through the cervical vertebrae and occipital bone. Because patients with recurring vertigo tend to be very anxious, physicians often assume they have psychosomatic problems and do not take them seriously. Unfortunately, this may simply increase the patient's anxiety, lead to further irritable or irrational behavior, reinforce the doctor's impression of a psychological problem, and so on in a vicious cycle. In this and many other cases, anxiety can magnify a small disorder into a large one. It is actually quite rare for a psychological problem to cause a positive Adson-Wright test. You should always search for physical explanations for the disturbance of arterial transit. Finally, do not confuse this type of vertigo with that of Ménière's disease; the latter disorder is also characterized by buzzing in the ears and deafness.

Problems of balance, which are less common than vertigo, are associated with similar positional changes, especially after waking up. *Ear problems* include earache, a sensation of the ear being blocked, or decreased hearing acuity.

Patients with inlet compression may report difficulty in waking up, mental fogginess, poor memory, and general malaise in the morning. Later in the day, these symptoms go away. The sleep of these patients has often been disturbed by nightmares. For this reason it is important to always check the inlets of children who frequently experience nightmares.

Finally, as mentioned above, thyroid problems or general thoracic or abdominal pain can also be related to compression of the inlet.

Neurological Problems

Because of their lateral location, the nerves of the thoracic inlet are influenced less than the blood vessels by mechanical problems of the cervicothoracic junction. They can be affected by direct or indirect trauma to the cervical spine or thorax. In this section, we will limit ourselves to describing disorders resulting from mechanical irritation of the vagus and phrenic nerves at the cervical or cervicothoracic level. While neurological paralysis and other problems due to trauma are also important, they fall outside the limits of this book and will not be discussed.

NEURITIS AND NEURALGIA

Neuritis (nerve inflammation) is associated with alteration or degeneration of nervous tissue, whereas neuralgia (pain felt along the course of a nerve) results from anatomical conditions and does not necessarily involve nerve tissue damage. Chest tightness and discomfort is likely to reflect a problem of the sympathetic nerves which rarely involves structural changes in the nerve itself. Therefore it is better if we only speak of neuralgia when discussing functional pains.

VAGUS NERVE DYSFUNCTIONS

Headache in this context is often related to sensory meningeal branches of the vagus nerve, which are distributed in the dura mater covering the ipsilateral cerebellar cavity, with some fibers going to the lateral and occipital sinuses. The area of the headache is fairly restricted and feels superficial to the patient. Osteopathic treatment is usually effective in these cases. However, we have had almost no success in treating "female" migraines. These headaches are associated with the menstrual cycle (they are usually worst just before the onset of the period), and disappear during pregnancy.

Some patients with vagus problems may experience sharp *precordial pain* around 4-5 AM. The patient wakes up for no apparent reason and feels the pain somewhat later. Precordial pain may also be triggered by activity with the arms in the air, intense exertion, or certain types of emotional upset. *Tachycardia,* occurring only during activity, but without other apparent cause, frequently accompanies precordial pain.

There may be *pain of the external auditory canal,* a tingling sensation, or general sense of discomfort in the ear. These patients may also report *pharyngeal pain,* irritation, or difficulty in swallowing, but examination of the throat shows nothing unusual. Cases of swallowing difficulty for which you cannot find any specific cause are dangerous, and should be referred quickly to a throat specialist.

Other symptoms of vagus dysfunction can be related to the gastric, hepatic, or esophageal branches, or to the celiac plexus. During our historical research, we were surprised to run across something called Thomas and Roux's sign of the celiac plexus, which we had noticed in our own treatments.

This sign, which had been essentially forgotten for about seventy years, is the disappearance of the radial pulse when pressure is applied to the epigastric fossa. This change is more significant when an abdominal organ is dysfunctional, making the celiac plexus more sensitive. This provides a good lesson on the importance of historical research for those of us who think we are innovators.

There are two vagal reflexes which can be easily tested. You should be familiar with these tests, which will help you recognize serious conditions that require referral to a specialist. The *velopalatin reflex,* elicited by stimulating the uvula or having the patient say "ah," consists of a lifting of the palate and symmetrical contraction of the faucial pillars. Its absence signifies injury to the medulla. The *gag reflex,* elicited by stimulating the posterior pharynx, consists of a contraction of the pharyngeal muscles and lifting of the soft palate. Its absence signifies injury to the vagus or glossopharyngeal nerve.

The vagus nerve sends out a recurrent nerve which encircles the inferior side of the subclavian artery. It is closely associated with the pleural dome and can be injured in pleuropulmonary disorders, causing, among other effects, laryngeal paralysis.

Recommendations: Be very careful when there is pain, partial anesthesia or paresthesia of the larynx, and discomfort with swallowing. The vagus is a complex nerve and its injury can cause a bewildering variety of neurological problems. This nerve supplies the smooth muscles of the digestive and respiratory system, and controls both cardiac rhythm and volume. It is the mediator for sensitivity and reflexes of all the viscera, controlling visceral sensations and our subconscious sense of visceral functions. With vagus disorders, this sense may rise to the conscious level. This condition, called cenesthesia, is very difficult for most patients to cope with.

SYMPATHETIC NERVOUS SYSTEM

Innervation

The sympathetic innervation of the thorax is mostly from the stellate ganglion and thoracic roots of the thoracic sympathetic nerves. The *stellate ganglion,* located on the anterior side of the transverse process of C7, represents the fusion of four or five cervical ganglia and one or two thoracic ganglia. Vascular branches from the stellate ganglion supply the vertebral and subclavian arteries and vertebrobasilar plexus. Visceral branches include fibers which supply the pleural dome and inferior cardiac nerves. In combination with the vagus nerve, the stellate ganglion forms coronary plexuses which supply the coronary arteries. This connection may explain certain coronary spasms associated with restrictions of the cervicothoracic junction.

Although we do not have solid proof, we suspect that the following clusters of symptoms can result from sympathetic dysfunction (there are, of course, other possible causes).

- Cardiac: arrhythmias, chest tightness and discomfort, anginal chest pain, and possibly coronary spasms.
- Circulatory: problems of the face, upper extremities, and superior thorax, often accompanied by abnormal sweating.
- Ocular: decreased visual acuity and miosis (contraction of the pupil). Cervicothoracic manipulations sometimes bring about an improvement of visual acuity which could be mediated via the sympathetic innervation of the eye. A patient presenting unilateral miosis associated with ipsilateral cervical restriction is a good candidate for osteopathic treatment. Sometimes, simple inhibition of the stellate ganglion reduces miosis.
- Digestive: This is the catch-all diagnosis for problems related to the digestive system which we are able to treat successfully. In our experience, it is essentially impossible to decide which problems are attributable to sympathetic versus parasympathetic dysfunction. On dissection, the nerves of these two systems appear hopelessly entangled with each other.
- Respiratory: another catch-all diagnosis, particularly for bronchospasms.

Sympathetic Trunk

The paired thoracic sympathetic trunk, which runs anterolaterally to the spinal cord, can cause a great variety of symptoms when restrictions are present. Look for cutaneous zones of different color and elasticity during physical exam. These often reflect a restriction of the corresponding vertebral segment. Sometimes there are false zoster-like eruptions, which last for several hours or days and then become painful (though less so than real herpes zoster) and a take on a darker skin color. Some so-called health practitioners are only too happy to claim success in treating herpes zoster when in fact they were dealing with a slight irritation of a sympathetic dorsal ganglion, which would probably have resolved by itself. With this type of symptom, one often finds a corresponding costovertebral restriction which responds well to manipulation.

Reflexes

The *pilomotor (or horripilation) reflex,* elicited by lightly tickling the neck, axilla, or infraclavicular area, consists of contraction of the arrector pili smooth muscles, with consequent elevation of the hairs and surrounding skin ("goose bumps"). Absence of this reflex suggests a lesion of the sympathetic trunk, plexus, peripheral nerves, or lateral horns of the medulla.

The *abdominal cutaneous reflexes* are tested using a fingernail, broken tongue depressor, etc., which is stroked across the surface of the abdomen toward the umbilicus. The normal reaction is a unilateral contraction of the abdominal muscles, pulling the umbilicus toward where you are stroking. The upper abdominal cutaneous reflex is tested approximately 4cm below the costal edge and evaluates spinal nerves T7-T9. The middle abdominal cutaneous reflex is tested lateral to the umbilicus and evaluates nerves T9-T11. The inferior abdominal cutaneous reflex is tested on a line parallel to but 4cm above the inguinal ligament and evaluates nerves T11-L1. Absence of these reflexes helps you to localize a problem at the spinal nerve level. They are also absent in diseases that affect the pyramidal tract, such as tabes dorsalis or multiple sclerosis.

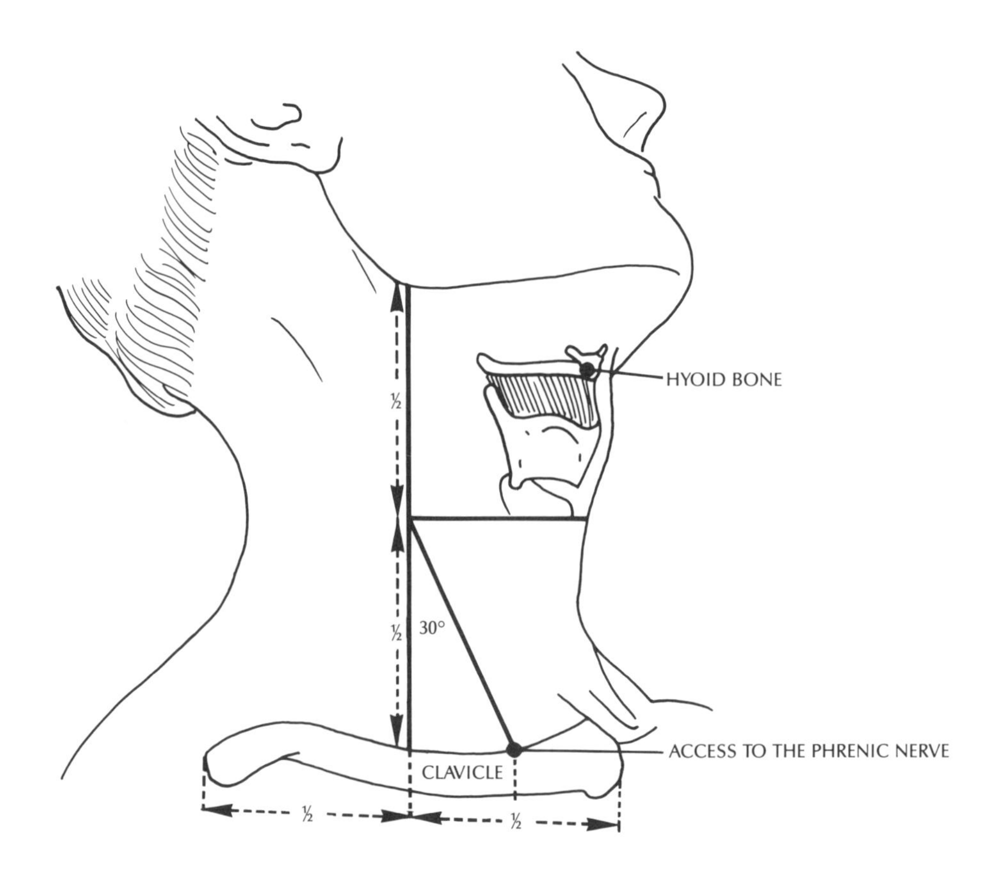

Illustration 5-5
Access to the Phrenic Nerve

PHRENIC NERVE

This nerve arises from the cervical plexus and supplies the diaphragm. Injury to the phrenic nerve is obvious in some cases (e.g., paradoxical respiration) but difficult to diagnose in others.

Trigger Points

There are many points that become tender or sore with phrenic problems, including C3-C4, the medial part of the intercostal spaces, and the anterior edge of rib 10. The phrenic nerve lies against the anterior face of the anterior scalene muscle. One particularly useful trigger point is found in the supraclavicular fossa and corresponds to the most accessible portion of the nerve, i.e., where the anterior scalene enters the triangular area bounded by the clavicle and the two heads of the sternocleidomastoid. To find this point, draw a line connecting the angle of the mandible to the middle of the clavicle. From the midpoint of this line, draw another line to the point halfway between the midpoint and medial end of the clavicle (Illustration 5-5). This second line should make an angle of 30 degrees with the first.

This trigger point, besides being very tender when the phrenic is irritated, is also useful for treating the lungs or diaphragm. For example, if you have difficulty improving the motility of the lung, gentle stimulation of this point will immediately help the process. Just posteromedial to this supraclavicular point is the vertebral artery. Gently stretching this area or inhibiting it can affect this artery and the blood supply to the posterior part of the brain, which can be helpful in cases of vertigo or loss of equilibrium.

Another important trigger point for the phrenic nerve is de Mussy's point, found at the intersection between an imaginary extension of the left sternal border and a transverse line at the level of the bony end of rib 10 (Illustration 5-6). This point is innervated by an abdominal branch of the phrenic nerve, and inhibition here affects all the organs supplied by the phrenic nerve. Our experience suggests that this point can also be used to release the subclavius muscle, which reflects the status of the phrenic nerve. For example, this muscle becomes exceedingly painful in cases with diaphragmatic pleuritis.

Both the trigger points described above are effective in specific situations. A thumb inhibiting the supraclavicular point works better in treating hiccups. De Mussy's point is more effective in stimulating the mobility and motility of the thoracic organs, gallbladder, and upper stomach.

Shoulder and elbow pain can also be due to disorders of the phrenic nerve, being mediated by branches of the C4 and C5 spinal nerves respectively. We have seen three cases of tennis elbow which did not respond to local manipulation and were eventually shown to be pain projected by a pulmonary condition.

Hiccups

This abrupt, involuntary, and rhythmic contraction of the diaphragm can result from cervical, mediastinal, or abdominal compression of the phrenic nerve, or from irritation of the nerve at the level of the pleura, mediastinum, pericardium, diaphragm, or peritoneum. In cases of chronic hiccups (we have seen several), refer the patient for a complete medical examination before beginning treatment. There is a possibility of tumor that must be ruled out.

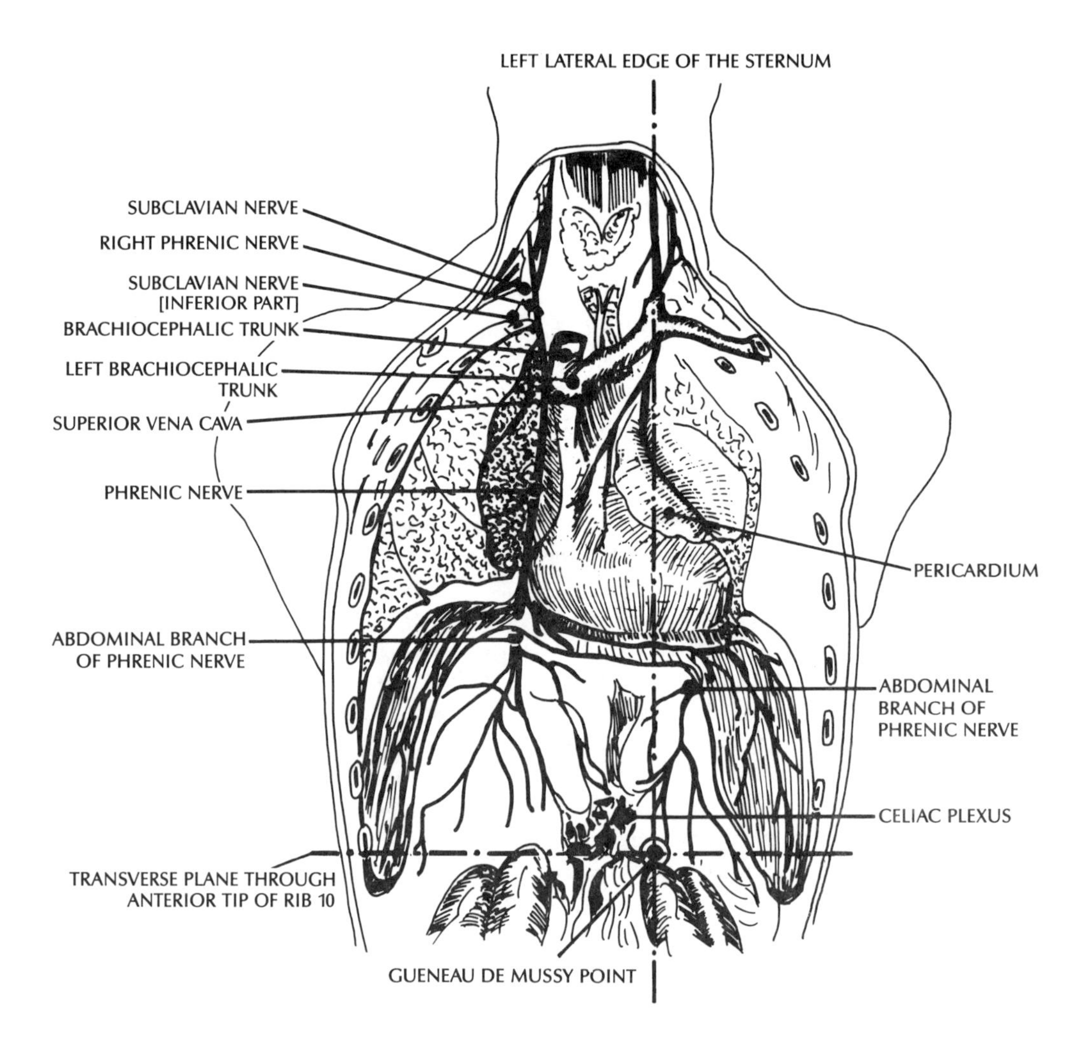

Illustration 5-6
De Mussy's Point

INTERCOSTAL NERVES

Intercostal nerves 1-6 provide sensory innervation to the anterolateral wall of the thorax. Nerves 4-6 also innervate the breast through extensions of their lateral and medial cutaneous branches called the lateral and medial mammary branches. Intercostal nerves 7-12 supply the peritoneum and abdominal wall.

Intercostal nerve 1 is the small branch of the first thoracic nerve, and is therefore related to the large branch of this spinal nerve, which ascends in front of the neck of rib 1 and contributes to the brachial plexus. This large branch is often connected to the stellate ganglion (injury to which causes Horner's syndrome; see below), and contains iridodilator fibers which supply the intrinsic muscular system of the eye. You should check this area in any patient with unilateral miosis.

Intercostal nerve 12 is actually subcostal. It sends off a lateral perforans branch which innervates the skin of the gluteal region and greater trochanter. Sometimes we see patients with trochanteric paresthesia who have negative radiological exams. This condition is usually the result of an old fall on the lower ribs and can be treated effectively by manipulation.

We have made an extremely rapid tour of the thoracic nervous system. As usual, we have confined ourselves to what we see in our daily practice. Before closing this section, we would like to warn you about the signs of *multiple sclerosis.* This is a progressive deterioration of myelin sheaths in the central nervous system and their replacement by sclerotic plaques. Initial diagnosis of this disease is extremely difficult. We have missed this diagnosis with patients who presented only with paresthesia of the thorax or legs. All examinations carried out at the time were negative and the correct diagnosis was made two or three years later. Be wary of isolated or multiple paresthesias associated with hyperreflexia and ocular, labyrinthine, or bladder symptoms. Particularly when recurrent, they are often the first signs of multiple sclerosis.

CERVICOBRACHIAL NEURALGIA

The nerve cords coming from the brachial plexus run posterosuperior to the subclavian artery. They occupy the posteroinferior angle of the supraclavicular fossa and are less affected by compression of the inlet than are blood vessels. Neuralgia in this area can have many causes, including the following.

With *degenerative joint disease of the cervical spine,* radiography reveals lipping of the vertebrae and narrowing of the vertebral foramina, mobility tests indicate a significant lower cervical restriction, and intertransverse pressure or craniocervical compression instantly recreates the pain. Be very wary of cervicobrachial neuralgia without osteoarticular restrictions, because these can be due to adenopathy of tumors as described below.

Cervicobrachial neuralgia often involves a *restriction of rib 1* (along with C7/T1) during inhalation. In this case, downward pressure on the first costovertebral junction will immediately trigger radicular pain. Adson-Wright test is often positive and ipsilateral systolic arterial pressure is low, possibly due to irritation of the stellate ganglion. Always check for miosis in these cases. Radicular pain of cervical or upper thoracic origin usually radiates to one or two fingers, or less commonly the whole hand. The fingers are either normally colored or pale. There is no edema or reddish coloring of the skin.

The cervicobrachial plexus can be also be compressed because of *adenopathy* due to problems of the face, neck, or thorax. You should know how to recognize adenopathies in the cervical, supraclavicular, and axillary regions. Troisier's node in the left supraclavicular fossa can be an indication of an abdominal lesion. Nodes in the right supraclavicular fossa are more likely to reflect problems of the thorax, face, or skull.

Tumors can be either mediastinal or pulmonary in origin (see Pancoast syndrome below).

NEUROLOGICAL SYNDROMES

Two neurological syndromes demonstrate the ability of nervous lesions to produce generalized symptoms. *Horner's syndrome,* due to an interruption of the cervical sympathetic chain, causes miosis, partial ptosis, enophthalmia (retraction of the eyeball into the orbit), vasomotor problems (often vasodilation), and absence of sweating on half of the face. There may also be decreased pilomotor response, problems in visual accommodation, or tachycardia. Etiology may be traumatic, vascular, tumoral, or adenopathic.

Pancoast syndrome, which occurs during the evolution of malignant tumors located near the pulmonary apex, includes pain which radiates to the shoulder, arm, and hand. It is more common on the left. Other neurologic manifestations can include paresis of the hand, fibrillations, and associated Horner's syndrome.

We have seen six patients who consulted us for cervicobrachial neuralgia shown to result from a pulmonary tumor. It seems strange to us that, while conventional physicians admit that reflex pain can be projected far from its origin in serious pathologies, they consistently deny the distant projections of pain which we see routinely in functional disorders.

Mobility Tests

This is a crucial section of the book, since only accurate mobility testing can enable us to choose the appropriate manipulative techniques. Skill in therapeutic manipulation without corresponding skill in diagnosis can be useless or even dangerous. At the beginning of Chapter 4, we mentioned the concept of the thorax as a "container" and the viscera as "contents." A restriction of the container has an effect on the contents, and vice versa. We will begin this section on mobility testing by discussing the container, then turn to the contents.

MECHANICAL THORACIC RESTRICTIONS

Deformation of the Thorax

The thorax is a complex structure containing more than 150 articulations, each of which will receive some part of the impact during falls and car crashes. Typically, the sternum receives the greatest part of the impact and then passes it on to the ribs, clavicles, viscera, etc. Some joints are able to make large movements, while others (e.g., cartilaginous joints) are more limited. Testing of the latter is just as important as the former. In our opinion, the difference between one osteopath and another lies in how detailed their concept of the body is and how specific their diagnostic and therapeutic abilities are.

All the thoracic fasciae are affected by deformation of the thorax. Consider a lung, which weighs about 1.3kg. In a fall or crash it will pull sharply on its upper attachments. These will absorb part of the shock, leading to cervical restrictions. The thorax, which some people think of as a mostly rigid unit, is in fact tremendously complex, containing over a hundred mobile elements, any of which may become restricted. Our job is to find these restrictions, wherever they may be.

Motor Vehicle Accidents

Twenty years ago when we began our practice, thoracic problems for which people consulted us were primarily due to direct trauma to the back, shoulders, or sternum, usually from falls. Some patients consulted for cervicothoracic pain resulting from pleuropulmonary conditions. Times have changed. While these problems still exist, automobile accidents have become the leading cause of thoracic restrictions in our patients.

The human body in a car crash suffers extraordinary pressures. It has been calculated that the "crash weight" of a man weighing 175 pounds whose vehicle comes to an abrupt stop from a speed of 55 miles per hour is nearly 2.5 tons (the weight of an elephant). Besides velocity and mass, actual duration of the crash affects the force to which the body is subjected. According to research done at the Volvo factory in Sweden, transmission of impact to the body in a typical head-on crash occurs within 2/25 of a second. This means the body and its organs absorb a huge force within a very brief period of time.

During a certain period following the accident, the victim is typically in shock. He may feel groggy and confused but not in significant pain. Progressively, in the days and weeks that follow, the pain appears—in the head, neck, sternum, ribs, etc. It is as if the different components of the body are releasing the force which they absorbed earlier, each in its own way. For example, the energy accumulated by a bone may be released intensely and quickly as a fracture. In contrast, effects of impact on soft tissues are less obvious. These tissues themselves only rarely rupture; while the force may slightly more often create slight osseous tears at their attachments, usually it stays in the tissues .

It is therefore the soft tissues that absorb most of the energy of a car crash. As they gradually heal themselves, they produce a variety of attendant symptoms. Since these symptoms are often subtle and difficult to explain, conventional physicians may ignore them, or glibly attribute them to post-traumatic depression or psychosomatic tendencies. Your responsibility as an osteopath is to carefully monitor the soft tissues over a long period of time by listening and mobility testing.

As mentioned in Chapter 1, we are aware that the seat belt saves many lives, but must point out that it also leads to numerous osteoarticular restrictions of the anterior thorax, particularly the sternoclavicular and acromioclavicular articulations and ribs. During a head-on crash, the force of the impact is concentrated around the seat belt, which holds back the bones and soft tissues immediately beneath it, while the rest of the thorax is pushed forward. Because of this peculiar situation, resulting thoracic restrictions can be quite complex. In cases of post-traumatic back pain, always test the anterior thorax; the cause may lie here.

Falls

Some falls, e.g., direct falls onto the shoulder, have obvious harmful effects on the acromial and sternoclavicular ligaments. However, many falls which appear trivial at the time can also lead to later problems. Falls onto the palm of the hand can create a sternoclavicular restriction which compresses the thoracic inlet. In many such cases, the patient does not even recall the incident. This is one of the reasons that we place greater reliance on what the tissues remember than on what the patient remembers. Interestingly, we have seen about ten cases of subluxation (partial dislocation) of the shoulder which happened during sleep to people with generally healthy muscle tone. This was probably due to relaxation of muscular tonus during vagal activity.

Fetal Position and Delivery

Obstetricians seldom worry about fetal position except in extreme cases, e.g., breech presentation, which can be seen by imaging techniques. We believe that sustained improper positioning, however slight, can cause contraction of the soft tissues leading to life-long problems. If you suspect that poor fetal position contributed to a present problem in a baby or small child, you need to find out exactly what the position was. For this, we utilize the memory of the fibers of the dura mater. With the patient in supine or seated position, push the skull gently in a caudal direction with one hand while the other pushes the sacrum cephalad. The amount of force used is slightly more than that used in craniosacral techniques. The spine will bend and rotate toward the position of ease, i.e., the fetal position. We have verified the accuracy of this test repeatedly by comparison with radiographs taken during the eighth month of pregnancy.

During delivery, thoracic injury to the baby is common when the head and arm emerge together. Some obstetricians, as long as there is no clavicular fracture, consider the delivery satisfactory. These people have no consideration of soft tissues. For example, we once assisted at a delivery which the obstetrician thought went very well. However, the baby was found to suffer from stretching of the brachial plexus with paresis of the arm. We must admit that obstetricians today are in general more sensitive and gentle than those of 15-20 years ago, and serious obstetrical injuries are becoming less frequent. It is a great challenge to the osteopath to recognize restrictions which appear in adolescence or adulthood but result primarily from something that happened during delivery. The medical history is usually not helpful in this situation. Apart from the obstetrician, the mother, and the patient's own tissues, who can evaluate the quality of delivery?

OSTEOARTICULAR TESTS

In the remainder of this chapter, we will describe the mobility tests we have developed in terms of four broad categories: osteoarticular, muscular, fascial, and visceral. We prefer to perform the osteoarticular tests in the seated position. This exposes muscular/ligamentous tensions which may be hidden when the patient is lying down. In addition, mobility tests should be synchronized with the rhythm of the patient's tissues for best results.

Sternoclavicular Joint

Sometimes we see patients who have real dislocations or subluxations of this joint. The restriction is so obvious that mobility tests are not necessary. You should not try to reposition this joint. After each attempt, the clavicle will return to its anterior position and your interference can irritate the cartilage and lead to a more serious chondritis. Even with a dislocation, however, a semblance of normal mobility can be restored. Always test both articulations, even if only one seems to be restricted; they are rendered interdependent by the interclavicular ligament.

For a test using compression/decompression, the patient sits in front of you, legs hanging down. One of your hands surrounds the shoulder (palm against the back) so that you can move it in any direction. One or two fingers of the other hand (testing hand) are placed on the sternoclavicular joint (Illustration 5-7).

The *posterior sternoclavicular ligament* resists posterior movement of the medial end of the clavicle. This is the ligament most affected in direct trauma to the sternum, or seat belt injuries. For testing, push the shoulder anteromedially, focusing the movement toward the sternoclavicular joint. With the thumb or index finger of the testing hand, accompany the posterior movement of the medial clavicle, accentuating it slightly. When there is a restriction, this movement becomes difficult or impossible. When the

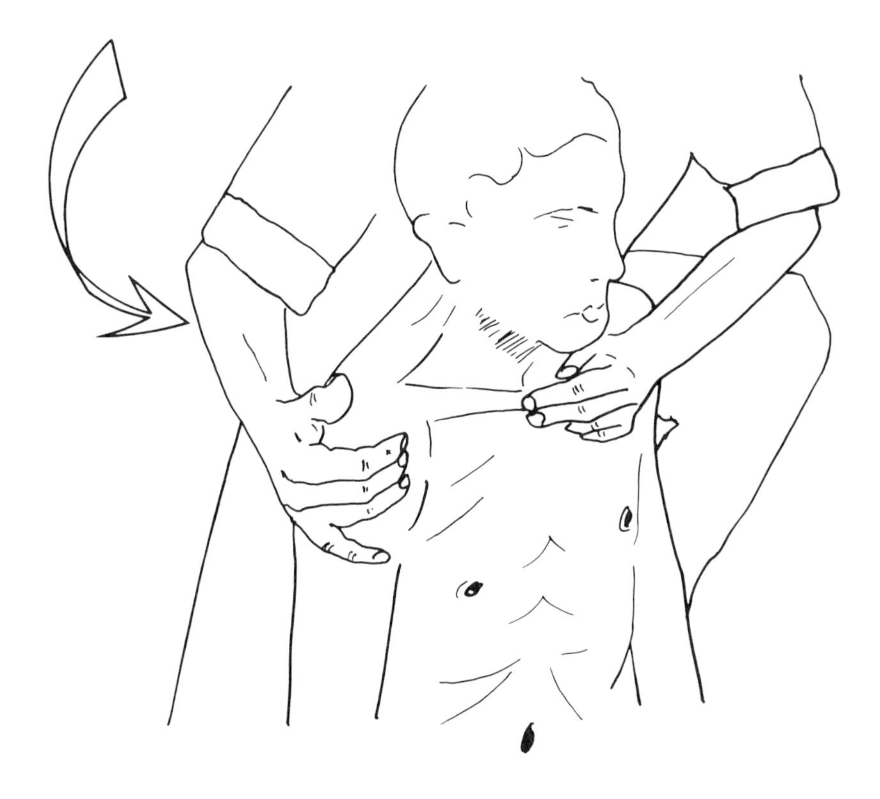

Illustration 5-7
Compression/Decompression Tests of the Sternoclavicular Joint

medial clavicle comes back slightly, pulled by the posterior ligament, you can also assess the anterior ligament.

The *anterior sternoclavicular ligament* resists anterior movement of the medial clavicle. This ligament (sometimes on both sides) is injured by falls onto the shoulder. In seat belt injuries, abrupt anterior movement of the clavicle creates a restriction of this ligament. Push the shoulder posterolaterally, until the medial clavicle moves forward. With the thumb or index finger of your testing hand, you can assess this anterior movement. With practice, you can test both anterior sternoclavicular ligaments at the same time.

The *interclavicular ligament* resists superior movement of the medial clavicle. It is commonly injured by falls onto the back, or when the thorax is pushed strongly anteroinferiorly. Push alternately on both shoulders, slightly posteriorly but primarily inferiorly, so that the medial clavicle moves upward. With the testing hand, you can monitor the existence and amplitude of the movement.

Acromioclavicular Joint

This is fixed with injury of the sternoclavicular joint or trauma to the shoulder. From our point of view, it is generally preferable to deal with a dislocation or even a fracture of the shoulder than ligamentous restrictions. The former are easier to diagnose, and treatment is usually more straightforward. With traumatic force not resulting in a dislocation, there are micro-ruptures and damage to joint capsules, muscles, and ligaments. Compared to dislocations, these are more difficult to diagnose, more complicated to treat, and slower to heal.

For a test using compression/decompression, the subject sits facing you with legs hanging down and the affected arm resting on your thigh in 90 degrees of abduction. One of your hands holds the shoulder while the testing hand pushes the lateral end of the clavicle inferiorly and slightly medially. In normal subjects, one feels the clavicle moving inferiorly and returning rapidly to its original position. With acromioclavicular problems, the movement is either too large or too small. You can test the anterior and posterior fibers separately by pushing the lateral clavicle anteriorly or posteriorly. To evaluate the joint itself, position the arm in abduction and external rotation. Place one finger of the testing hand on the lateral clavicle to evaluate movement at the joint as the other hand moves the forearm alternately frontward and backward.

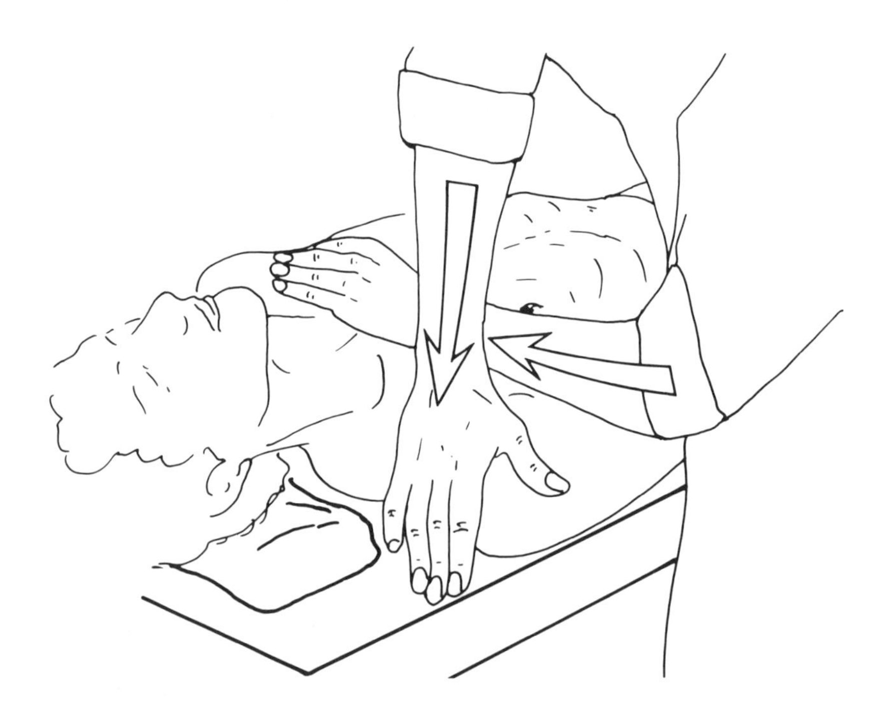

Illustration 5-8
Conoid and Trapezoid Ligament Tests

Ligaments of the Coracoid Process

When the arm is hanging down, the coracoid process is found at the top of the deltopectoral groove, 2.5cm below the junction of the lateral and middle thirds of the clavicle. To test the *trapezoid ligament* with the patient in seated position, press the coracoid with the thumb of the testing hand while the other pushes the lateral clavicle superolaterally. This ligament can also be tested in the supine position, with your hands crossed over. Place your two hypothenar eminences (or thumbs) on the coracoid and clavicle and stretch the ligament by pushing in different directions. For the trapezoid the force on the clavicle goes superolaterally, while that on the coracoid goes inferomedially (Illustration 5-8). To test the *conoid ligament,* press the medial part of the coracoid with the thumb of the testing hand while the other pushes the middle clavicle posterosuperiorly and medially. Testing of these two coracoclavicular ligaments is difficult at first, but becomes easier with practice. Always compare the ligaments with their counterparts on the opposite side. The lateral part of the subclavius muscle is closely associated with these ligaments, so restrictions are usually shared.

For testing of the *acromiocoracoid ligaments,* with the patient in lateral decubitus or supine position, press posteriorly with the testing hand on the acromion and push posteromedially on the coracoid with the palm of the other hand (Illustration 5-9). You cannot evaluate these ligaments very precisely (as you can, for example, the anterior sternoclavicular ligament) because they normally function as an osteofibrous dome. Simply evaluate their general elasticity. When restricted, they can interfere with the articular interplay of the shoulder girdle.

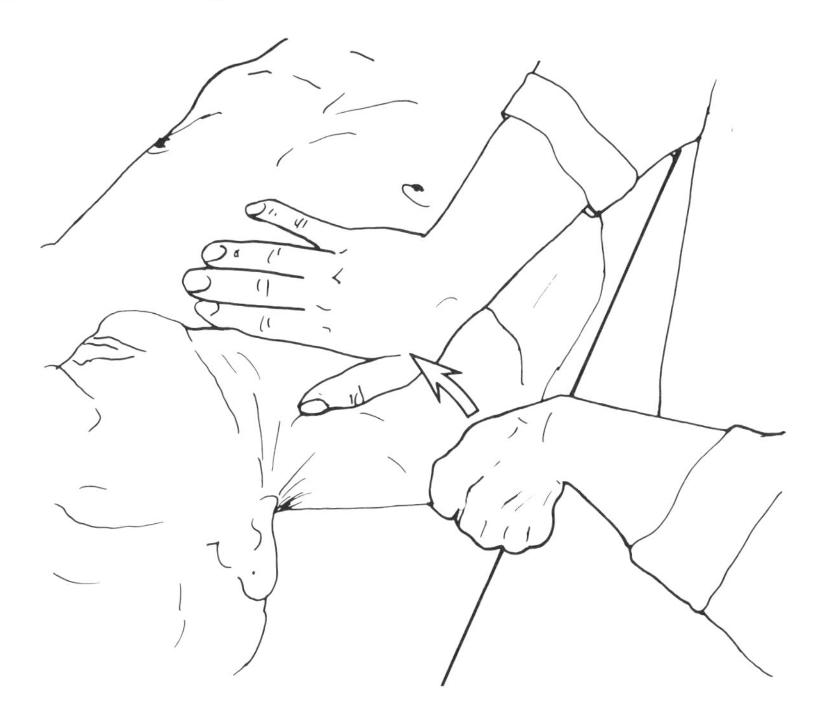

Illustration 5-9
Acromiocorocoid Ligament Tests

Longitudinal Clavicular Compression

This is a general test that with one movement checks for any clavicular restrictions. This can be done in the supine, lateral decubitus, or seated positions. We prefer the supine position. One hypothenar eminence is placed on the clavicular aspect of the sternoclavicular joint. The other hypothenar eminence is on the clavicular aspect of the acromioclavicular joint. They simultaneously press toward each other (Illustration 5-10). When there is a restriction of the clavicle, it lacks the normal elasticity. You then have to analyze whether the resistance comes from the middle, lateral, or medial part of the clavicle.

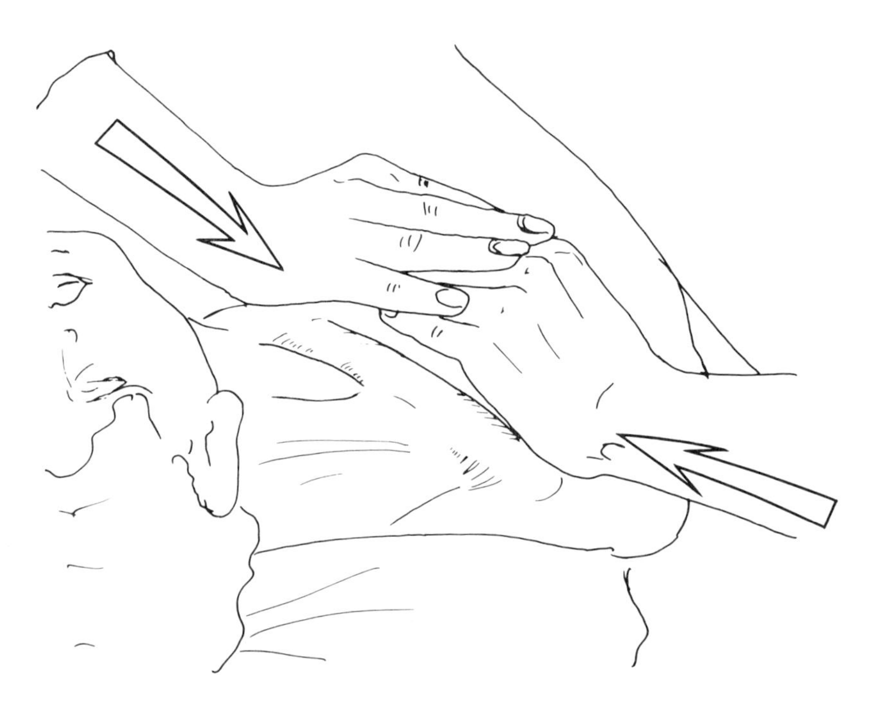

Illustration 5-10
Longitudinal Clavicular Compression

Sternum

This strong, flat bone receives all the mechanical tensions of the thorax. There are intrasternal joints as well as articulations with the ribs. The following *compression/decompression test* can also be used for diagnosis of deeper visceral/mediastinal restrictions. This test is similar to the uterosacral test applied via the sacrum, i.e., you start by pressing the bone posteriorly and evaluate the resistance. You then release the pressure and evaluate how quickly and smoothly the bone returns to its anterior position. Perform this test first at the sternal angle and then between the angle and the xiphoid process. If compression is difficult, concentrate on checking for sternochondral restrictions where the sternum moves the least. If compression is easy but return is slow, look for mediastinal or pericardial tensions. You should test not only the three parts of the sternum itself but also all the sternochondral joints and attached soft tissues (pericardium, pleura, etc.) Practice on patients with documented pleural or pericardial problems to familiarize yourself with the associated difficulty in return. Because of the presence of the heart, mobility is more limited with sternal compression on the left side.

Another mobility test called the *sternal lift* is a useful technique for the entire pericardial/pleural/mediastinal system, although it is sometimes difficult to perform.

Place the index fingers of both hands like hooks, against or under the sternal notch and xiphoid process respectively. Pull lightly with both fingers to move the sternum anteriorly (Illustration 5-11). In contrast to direct tests (which have very clear barriers), you will feel the sternum go into "listening" during this test. Your hands feel as if they are moving a long way and floating slowly; during this process they will slide very subtly toward the area of restriction. We suggest that you try out this test to feel the sternal sliding in listening, and compare it to the movement you feel on joint testing.

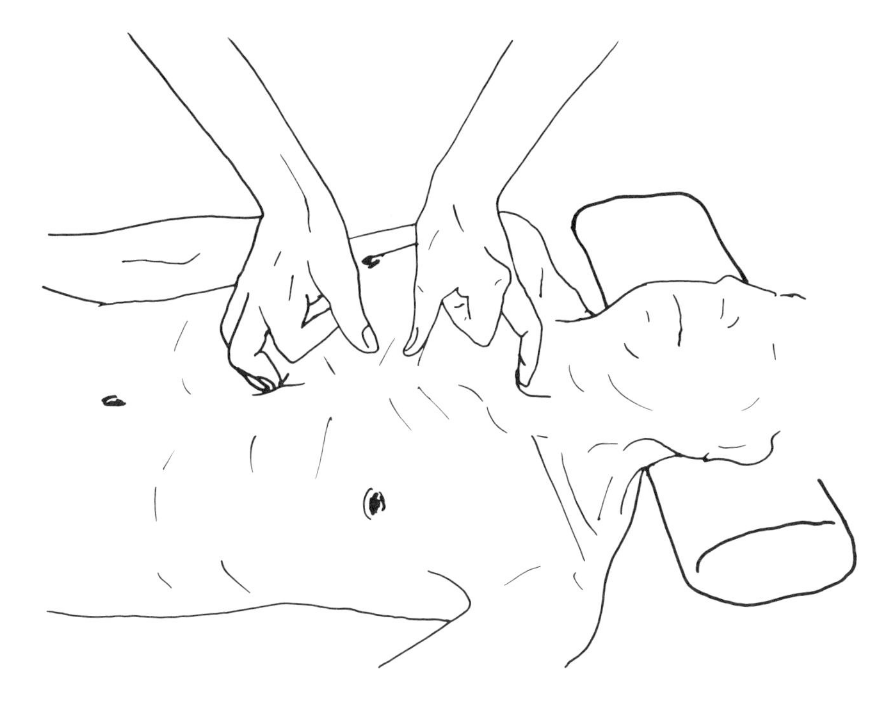

Illustration 5-11
Sternal Lift

Intrasternal Joints

Effects of trauma are often concentrated around the superior sternum and second sternochondral articulations. Restrictions here cause local pain and limit deep inhalation. A test of the *sternomanubrial joint* is performed by placing one palm on the manubrium, very close to the sternoclavicular joints, and the other on the sternal body just below the angle. Push your palms together as if trying to make the angle protrude (Illustration 5-12). A simpler method is to press the palm of one hand on the angle to evaluate the elasticity of the joint. We prefer to use the first method when possible because it gives more information.

A test of the *sternoxiphoid joint* consists of pushing anterosuperiorly on the xiphoid process with one finger to assess its elasticity. This technique is difficult for beginners. You do not need to put your finger behind the xiphoid; just press the finger against the inferior border and push superiorly to get some compression. This may be sufficient to find a restriction. Alternatively, leave the finger on the inferior xiphoid and push the

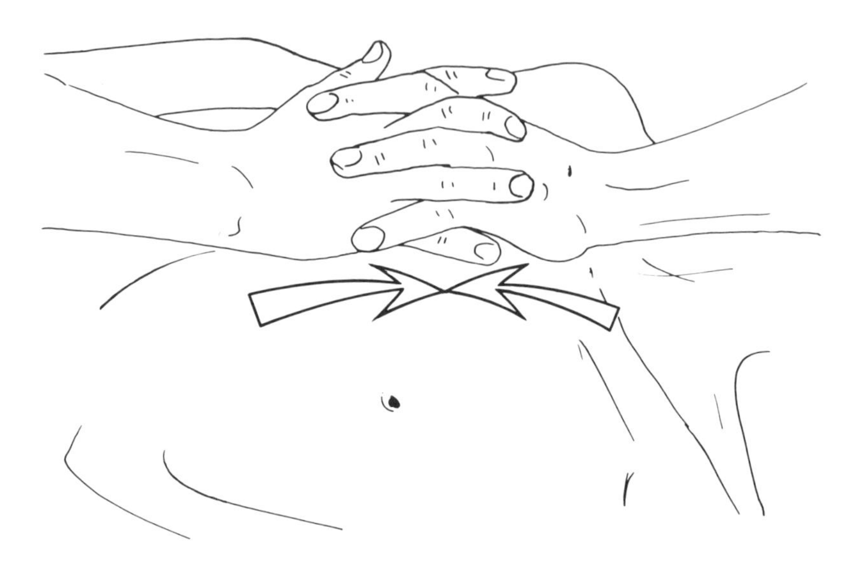

Illustration 5-12
Sternomanubrial Test

rest of the sternum inferiorly against it. If there is a restriction of the sternoxiphoid joint, you will feel a sidebending or rotation. It is common to find simultaneous injuries to the inferior sternum and seventh sternochondral joints resulting from direct frontal trauma (such as a blow from a fist, impact with dashboard, or falling down flat on the stomach).

Sternovertebral Test

This is similar to the compression/decompression test for the sternum described above. It is a general test of the soft tissues between the sternum and T4, especially the mediastinum and pleura. We can conceptualize the mediastinum as a bag going from the thoracic spine to the sternum. This test should be performed with the patient in seated position because some restrictions are more obvious this way than with the supine position. Place one palm against the spinous processes of T4-T5 and the other on the sternal body. With the anterior hand, apply a slight posterior pressure to the sternum that causes it to slide (e.g., from bottom to top or right to left). The posterior hand acts as a stabilizer and aids in focusing. Both the amount of force used in this test and the amplitude of the motion being tested are between normal mobility tests and listening.

Sternochondral and Costochondral Joints

It is a pity that the anatomists who write textbooks are not osteopaths. Then they would be aware of all the movements of which articulations of the human body are capable. Obviously, certain articulations in a dead body appear immobile, as we have verified many times. In a living, functioning body the situation is very different. As a case in point, the sternochondral and costochondral joints have significant mobility, and are affected by direct trauma or falls on the shoulder. These joints participate in every respiratory or other movement of the thorax, so restrictions here are critical.

Compression/decompression tests of the sternochondral joints can be carried out in seated or supine position. For the test in seated position, use one hand to bring the shoulder anteromedially (for compression) and posterolaterally (for decompression). Place one or two fingers of the testing hand on the sternochondral joints in order to feel the mobility of the costal cartilages on the sternum (Illustration 5-13). With compression, the anteromedial movement of the shoulder brings the cartilage into a posterior position in relation to the sternum. You can increase this tendency with your finger. With a restriction there will be a sensation of hardness and pain with pressure (note: pain on pressure does not occur with fibrous joints). With decompression, you let the cartilage return anteriorly, while mobilizing the shoulder posterolaterally, and evaluate the return with the finger of the testing hand. We prefer the compression test because it is easier to feel, and also accompanied by pain when there is a restriction, which makes it virtually impossible to miss.

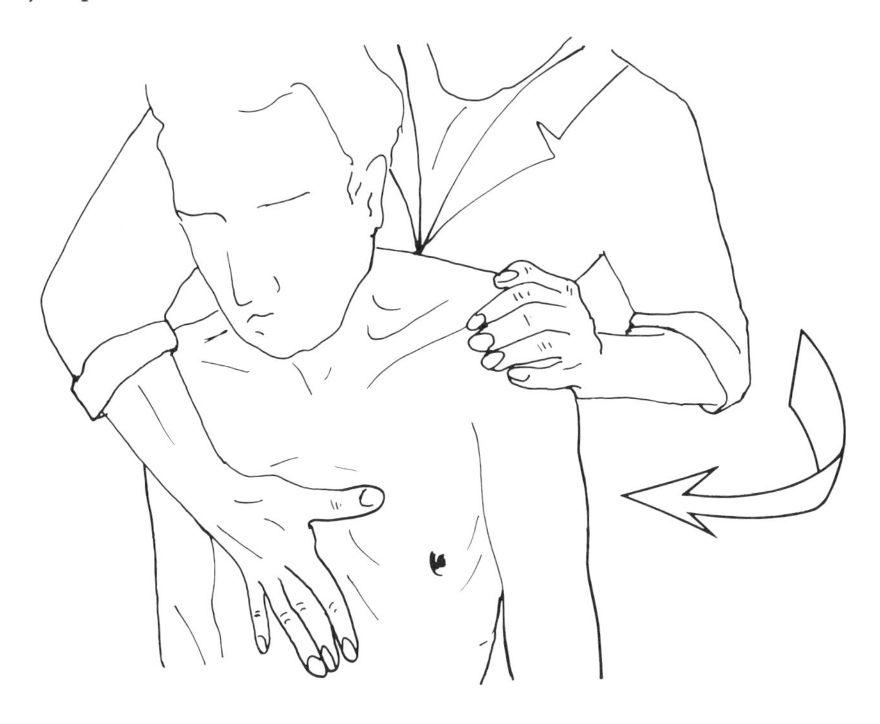

Illustration 5-13
Sternochondral Test in the Seated Position (Compression)

For the alternative sternochondral test in the supine position, use one hand to stretch the arm on the side to be tested anteriorly and slightly medially. With the thumb of the testing hand, put posterior pressure on the cartilage of the joint in question (Illustration 5-14). This test can easily be modified to become a treatment, as explained in the next chapter.

When testing the first sternochondral joint, you must also check its relation to the clavicle. This will be discussed below in connection with the test for the subclavius muscle, as restrictions of this muscle and the first sternochondral always occur simultaneously.

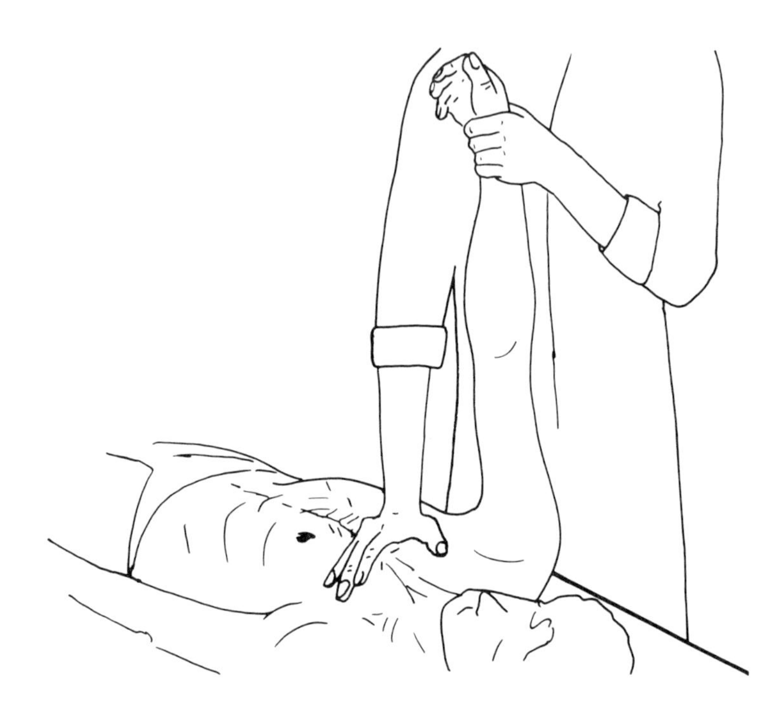

Illustration 5-14
Sternochondral Test in the Supine Position (Compression)

Tests for the *costochondral joints* are very similar to those for the sternochondrals. The fingers are placed on the costochondral junctions, which are located about two finger-widths lateral to the sternochondrals. These joints are important since they can cause chronic intercostal restrictions with potential effects on the pleura.

MUSCULAR TESTS

We will not discuss the large thoracic muscles (e.g., pectorals, deltoids), which do not present chronic pathogenic restrictions. Acute spasms of these muscles are always secondary and resolve spontaneously. Certain smaller muscles, for which tests are described below, are ignored by many practitioners of manual medicine. Since manipulation of these smaller muscles can give good results in some cases, you should be familiar with appropriate diagnostic methods. We generally prefer passive tests to active tests (in which the patient is asked to inhale or to contract certain muscles); our experience has shown the passive tests to allow greater precision. Also, it is usually easier to evaluate all the fibers when the patient is passive.

Subclavius

This muscle originates at the medial end of rib 1 and runs superolaterally and posteriorly to insert under the clavicle. It can be tested in either the seated, supine, or lateral decubitus positions. The costoclavicular ligament and first sternochondral joint can be tested at the same time. The only way to differentiate between problems of the costoclavicular ligament and the subclavius is by direct palpation. The ligament is found at the most medial aspect of the space between the clavicle and rib 1, and of course feels firmer. This distinction is largely hypothetical because these two structures are almost always restricted, and can be treated, together. The conoid and trapezoid ligaments (see under "Osteoarticular Tests" above) exchange fibers with the subclavius, and must also be tested when a restriction is found here.

For testing in the seated position, place the thumb of the testing hand inferomedially on rib 1 and press it against its sternochondral joint. Place the fingers of the other hand against the medial anteroinferior part of the clavicle and lift it superolaterally. You will feel more of an impression of elasticity than an actual movement. Always compare both sides.

For testing in the supine position, lift the patient's arm on the side to be tested anteriorly and then slightly medially. Alternately, the hand is placed by the patient's side and the shoulder is brought anteromedially. The thumb of the testing hand presses rib 1 posterolaterally (Illustration 5-15). You should feel a sensation of elasticity as well as some actual movement.

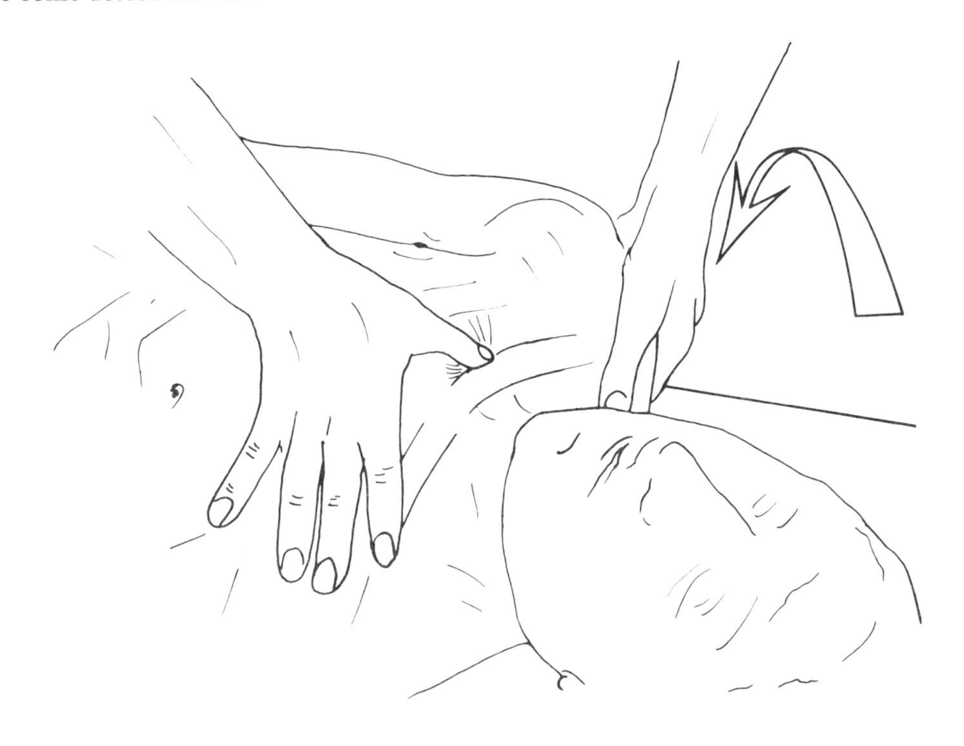

Illustration 5-15
Subclavius Muscle Test in the Supine Position

For testing in the lateral decubitus position, the patient lies on his side facing you. With one hand, move the shoulder anteriorly and slightly medially, focusing the movement on the clavicle. Your testing hand holds rib 1 in place, or pushes it slightly posteriorly. This method lets you evaluate both movement and elasticity of the subclavius.

Another test for evaluating muscular tension is performed with the patient in the same position. Place your thumb underneath the anterior part of the clavicle, while your index finger curls around the back of the clavicle and presses in deeply (Illustration 5-16). This pinching action allows you to directly check both the mobility and tension of the subclavius.

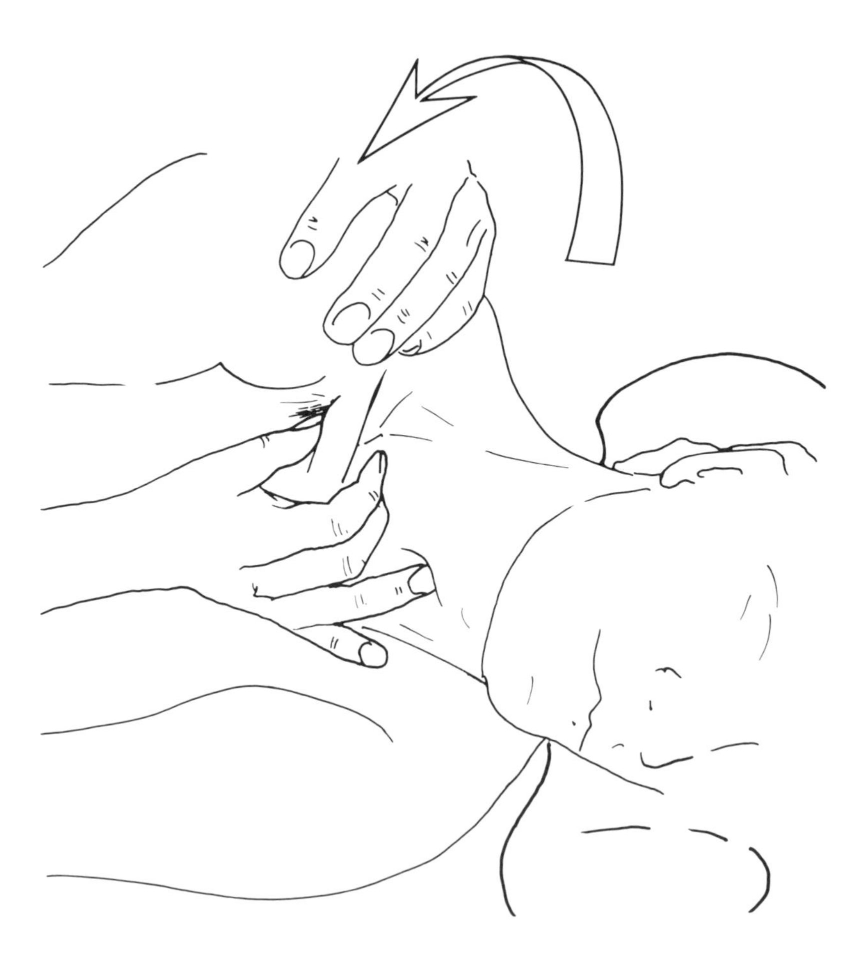

Illustration 5-16
Pinching the Subclavius Muscle

Transversus Thoracis

Specific testing of this muscle can be difficult or impossible in some patients, although its treatment is relatively simple. It originates on the posterior surface of the sternum and xiphoid, and inserts on costal cartilages 2-6. The fibers run inferomedially. This muscle can be injured by sternocostal traumas or pleural conditions. Testing it involves pushing the sternum posteroinferiorly. With a restriction, there is considerable resistance, often combined with rotation or sidebending of the sternum. However, a variety of lower sternal restrictions can give this same finding.

Intercostals

The *external intercostal muscles* occupy mostly the posterior and anterolateral parts of the intercostal spaces. They are usually restricted following costal trauma. Testing can be performed in seated or supine position. In the seated position, the patient clasps his hands behind the head, and you stand behind him, one foot resting on the table. Hold the elbows in one hand and use them to bring the thorax into backward bending to the level desired, then sidebend and rotate the trunk toward the side opposite the ribs to be tested. The thumb of the testing hand pushes the ribs anteroinferiorly to evaluate intercostal movement (Illustration 5-17). Bend the vertebral column farther and farther backward to focus on the descending levels of the muscles. The lateral portion of the external intercostals is tested in the same position but the sidebending is carried out without rotation, toward the side of the ribs to be tested. The thumb moves the ribs inferomedially. These muscles stop at the level of the costochondral joints. To test the anterior portion of the muscles with the patient in this position, push the thumb of the testing hand anteriorly against the superior edge of a rib to move it inferomedially, while bending the thorax forward and backward to focus the movement on the appropriate intercostal space.

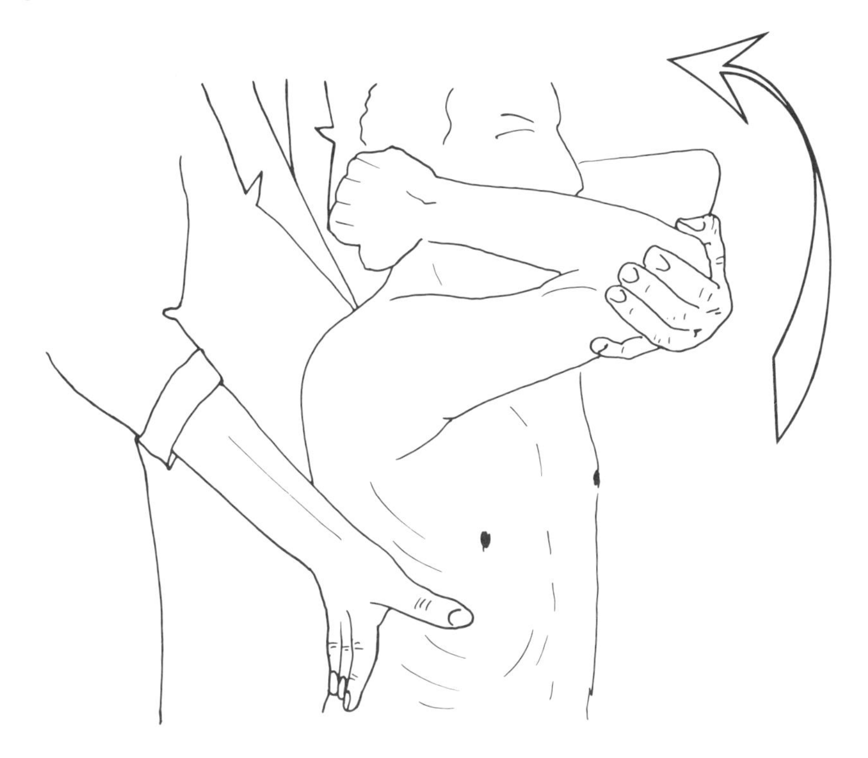

Illustration 5-17
Test of the External Intercostal Muscles (Posterior Part): Seated Position

For testing the external intercostals in the supine position, stand behind the patient's head or shoulder on the side of the muscle to be tested. Use both thumbs to push the ribs inferomedially and slightly posteriorly. Alternatively, lift the ipsilateral arm upward (shoulder flexion) and medially with one hand, while pushing inferomedially with the testing hand against the upper edge of the ribs.

We rarely try to perform specific mobility tests for the *internal intercostal muscles.* Their restrictions are difficult to distinguish from those of the external intercostals, as both prevent the inferior edge of a rib from separating from the superior edge of the rib below. The internal intercostals do not extend past the posterior angle of the ribs. They can be tested in the supine position using a method similar to that for the external intercostals, except that the ribs have to be pushed posteroinferiorly and laterally. When an external intercostal is restricted, the corresponding internal intercostal will generally also be restricted. There is a close relationship between the internal intercostals and the pleura. Trauma to the ribs can cause a pleural restriction, and vice versa. The subcostal muscles are not distinguished from the intercostal muscles in terms of testing and treatment.

Levatores Costarum

These muscles are often fixed in cases of very old thoracic injury. They originate on the transverse processes and insert on the angle of the rib one or two segments below. For the test in the seated position, have the patient sit in front of you with both hands behind his head. Raise his two elbows with one of your hands, rotating the torso toward the side opposite the muscles to be tested. Place the thumb of the testing hand on the posterior angle of the rib, and push the rib inferolaterally, away from the transverse process above. When there is a restriction, it is very difficult to move the posterior angle in this direction.

For the test in the prone position, have the patient lie flat on his stomach, head rotated toward the side opposite the muscles to be tested. Place one palm on the posterior angle of the rib, pushing it inferolaterally, while the other palm stabilizes the transverse process above by pressing anteriorly and toward the opposite side. Normally you will feel an elasticity rather than an actual movement.

Diaphragm

Basically, we do not believe that there are primary restrictions of the diaphragm. Apparent restrictions of this muscle invariably reflect some emotional, visceral, or articular problem. In testing the diaphragm, you should be careful about diagnosing a lateral predominance as pathological. This phenomenon (i.e., one side being stronger than the other) applies to the left versus right hemidiaphragm just as it does to most of the paired structures (such as the eyes, ears, or arms).

Emotional restrictions of the diaphragm are **bilateral** and limit its mobility, preventing deep inhalation. The patient gets out of breath very quickly, and has a tendency to spasmophilia. In local listening, the palm of the hand moves toward the celiac or cardiac plexus. Inhibition of the plexuses produces a temporary release of these restrictions. The patient is often hyperreflexive and shows Chvostek's sign (spasm of the ipsilateral facial muscles when the area in front of the ear is tapped). This sign is not specific for tetanus or hypocalcemia (as is sometimes stated), but is often found with general anxiety or chronic colitis.

Visceral restrictions of the diaphragm are **unilateral** and usually correspond to malfunction of a particular organ suspended from the diaphragm. For example, a heavier-than-normal liver will pull on its phrenic attachments, limiting the movement of the right hemidiaphragm. Glisson's capsule and part of the perihepatic peritoneum are innervated by the phrenic nerve, and irritation of this nerve in this situation can create spasms and limited mobility of the right hemidiaphragm. Local listening brings the palm against the liver, and an inhibition technique during inhalation will immediately restore normal mobility. Of course, when the pleura is restricted on one side, that hemidiaphragm will also be restricted.

There are numerous possible *osteoarticular restrictions* of the diaphragm. They are usually unilateral. Cervical problems affect the diaphragm via the phrenic nerve and the suspensory ligaments of the pleura. The ribs affect the diaphragm via the pleura and its diaphragmatic attachments. The vertebrae of the thoracolumbar junction affect it via the attachments of the pillars of the diaphragm, and by various nervous pathways. These causes can be identified by general and local listening.

FASCIAL TESTS

Testing and manipulation of the fasciae are important in terms of the respiratory and circulatory systems. It is possible to directly stretch the fasciae, notably inside the rib cage using a retroclavicular route. The fascial system is typically affected by cervicothoracic trauma and disorders of the heart, pleura, or lungs. We believe that, like the muscular system, it "memorizes" the forces experienced during major traumas.

Middle Cervical Aponeurosis

Testing of this structure utilizes the tension of the omohyoid and infrahyoid muscles. It is helpful to stabilize the hyoid bone and stretch the middle cervical aponeurosis by pushing inferiorly in turn on the clavicle, rib 1, and scapula. We have found stabilization of the hyoid to be much easier in the supine than in the seated position. The superficial cervical aponeurosis is too thin to produce genuine restrictions. The infrahyoid muscles are tested similarly to the middle cervical aponeurosis; their restrictions tend to be less pathogenic.

For a test in the *supine position,* have the patient lie down with both arms along his body. Stabilize the hyoid with the thumb and index finger (or index and middle fingers) of one hand, and use the thumb and heel of the other hand to push sequentially on several bony structures and associated soft tissues. Pressure is placed first on the clavicle and rib 1, focusing on the medial clavicle. Next, press on the middle clavicle, and finally the superomedial scapula (Illustration 5-18). A restriction is revealed by a relative lack of distensibility of the middle cervical aponeurosis, which can sometimes be observed with the naked eye during this test. Always compare both sides.

The motion of these structures should first be appreciated during normal breathing. If the hyoid is pulled down on one side, usually a thoracic restriction is the cause; if it is pulled up, the restriction is usually in the skull. The motion testing described above is best carried out during exhalation.

Alternatively, have the patient rotate and sidebend his head toward the side opposite that to be tested and rest it on your abdomen or thigh. Spread the fingers of your testing hand widely across the space between the hyoid bone and clavicle, while the other hand pushes the clavicle in an inferolateral direction. Simultaneously, use your abdomen to

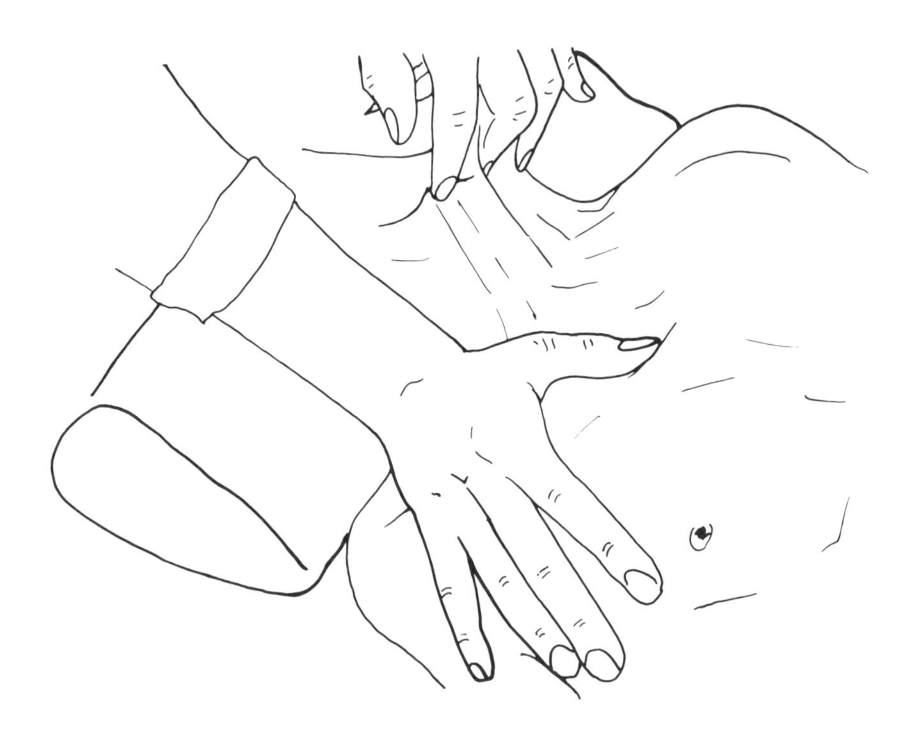

Illustration 5-18
Test of the Middle Cervical Aponeurosis: Supine Position

rotate and slightly sidebend the head toward the opposite side. This test sounds complicated, but is easy to carry out. A variation of the test in this position involves fixing various parts of the middle cervical aponeurosis with one thumb, e.g., deep in the supraclavicular fossa, on the scapula, on rib 1, etc. With your abdomen, carry out stretching movements focused on the part being fixed. This method permits precise localization of the restriction.

For a test of the middle cervical aponeurosis in the *seated position,* the patient sits with his back against you. Use one hand to stretch the head and cervical spine into sidebending rotation toward the side opposite that to be tested. The thumb of your testing hand fixes the middle cervical aponeurosis successively on its lateral, middle, and medial parts (Illustration 5-19). To test the medial part, you must first fix it against the posterior aspect of the sternoclavicular joint, and then push it posteroinferiorly to increase the tension. Some might criticize this test on the grounds that it also tenses the scalene muscles. However, it is easy to differentiate between the tension of an aponeurosis versus a muscle. The middle cervical aponeurosis, which is only a thin layer of tissue, feels flat and light. The muscle feels round and thicker. It you have any doubt, have the patient turn his head against pressure. You will feel the contraction of the muscle immediately; this makes it easy to distinguish the tension of the aponeurosis from that of the muscle.

Clavipectoral Fascia

This fascia inserts into the coracoid process, brachial aponeurosis, and aponeurosis of the subclavius muscle. For testing, place the patient in supine position, with the

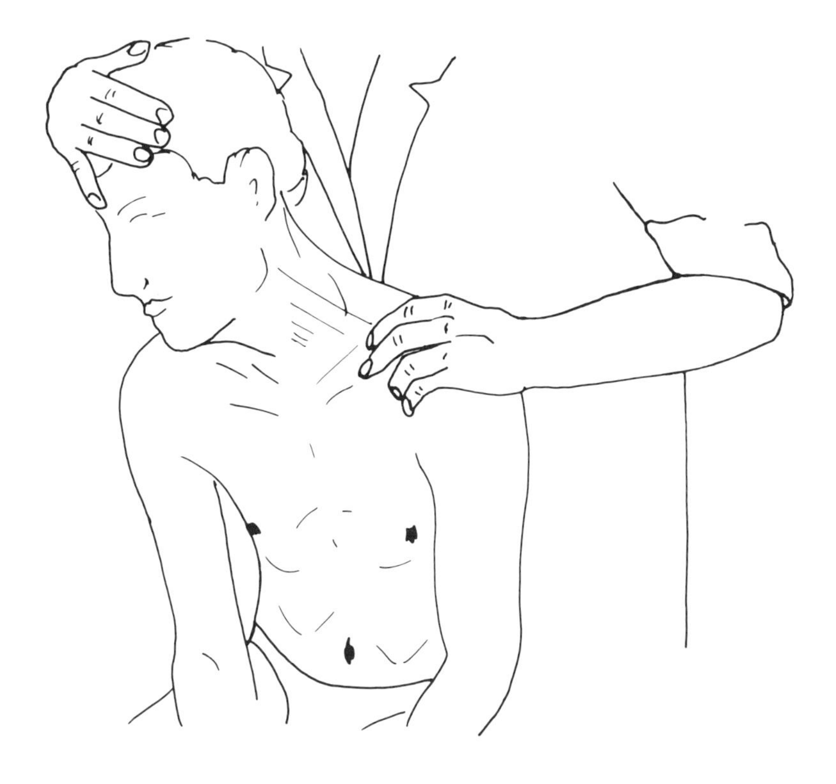

Illustration 5-19
Test of the Middle Cervical Aponeurosis: Seated Position

head sidebent and rotated toward the side opposite that to be tested, and ipsilateral arm lying on the table in abduction and external rotation. To test the origin, rotate and sidebend the head toward the contralateral side to fix the clavicle and middle cervical aponeurosis (which exchanges fibers with the clavipectoral). To test the insertion, abduct and externally rotate the arm a full 90 degrees to fix the brachial aponeurosis, where the clavipectoral ends. Press the palm of one hand against the anteroinferior part of the clavicle, while the other palm pushes the coracoid process inferolaterally. It is easier if you have your arms crossed and use the hand on the clavicle to push it superomedially at the same time. Compare both sides. With a significant restriction of the clavipectoral, this movement is difficult and the patient feels a sensation of uneasiness or oppression. With practice, you will be able to perform this test replacing pressure on the clavicle with lateral cervical pressure, which induces tension of the middle cervical aponeurosis and thus, indirectly, the clavipectoral.

Pleura

This fascia surrounds the lungs. It would obviously be impractical to try to test it everywhere, but experience has shown us that three parts have the greatest diagnostic significance: the cervicopleural suspensory apparatus, costomediastinal recesses, and costodiaphragmatic recesses. We have a preference for the former because it can be palpated directly and often shows positive results on manipulation. The pleura can be injured by any pleuropulmonary disorder or thoracic trauma, even by activities involving movement of the arms against resistance. Such injuries can cause recurrent cervical pain; symptoms may subside for several days after manipulation, but then reappear.

Cervicopleural Suspensory Apparatus

This fascia runs from cervical vertebrae 6-7 to ribs 1-2. The insertions are next to the scalene tubercle, which is why we use the lower point for pressure. There are several possible tests. We prefer the *passive test in the seated position* because in it gravity plays its usual role and the lung exerts its usual traction. The patient sits against you, his arm resting on your knee. Place the thumb of your testing hand deeply behind the clavicle, against the scalene tubercle. With the other hand, rotate and sidebend the head toward the opposite side until you feel the cervicopleural fibers stretch under your fingers. Use the thumb to evaluate the various fibers running from the cervical spine up to rib 1 by moving it in the direction of the neck of this rib, where the costopleural ligament inserts. Be alert for subcutaneous crepitation, which can signify a pneumothorax. The patient may cough because of irritation to the phrenic nerve and pleural stimulation. With a restriction of the cervicopleural suspensory apparatus, you will feel thickened fibers which are difficult to mobilize, and the patient will report discomfort on inhalation. This test can also be done by playing on the different suspensory fibers like guitar strings. By comparing their elasticity, you can rapidly identify specific areas of restriction.

For an *active test in the seated position,* maintain the thumb against rib 1 and ask the patient to inhale more deeply. With a restriction, you will feel significant fascial tension under your thumb, while the patient will report tension in the chest and respiratory discomfort. During inhalation, push the anterior surface of the rib toward the arm. A cervical or sternochondral articular restriction gives the impression of a hard, osseous barrier, whereas with a cervicopleural restriction the movement is reduced but still present.

For a *test in the supine position,* the patient lies with his head resting on your abdomen. Place both thumbs inside the supraclavicular fossae, one against the scalene tubercle, the other more posteriorly, against the neck of rib 1. Use your abdomen to sidebend the head to both sides, and successively evaluate the various pleural attachments on both sides. The technique can also be performed with one thumb in each supraclavicular fossa (Illustration 5-20). This test is useful in that it allows direct comparison of both sides and brings the cervical spine into play without effort. The thumbs can evaluate cervicopleural distensibility by playing on the various fibers like guitar strings.

For a *test in the lateral decubitus position,* the patient lies on the side to be tested, upper leg bent, other leg extended for balance. Clasp one hand around the shoulder to draw it inferomedially, and use the thumb of your testing hand as described above to deeply explore the tensions of the suspensory apparatus. Since in this position the neck is already sidebent, all you need to do is slightly rotate the head toward the contralateral side. This test allows the deepest penetration, in part because sidebending is the most prominent motion used (in this area, rotation usually involves more superficial tissues). Also, the thumb is able to evaluate all the fasciae in the supraclavicular fossa (including the more posteriorly located) by pressing against the neck of rib 1.

Costomediastinal Recesses

The insertions of these structures are fairly complex, but our experience has shown that their restrictions are focused around the fourth sternochondral joints. In the

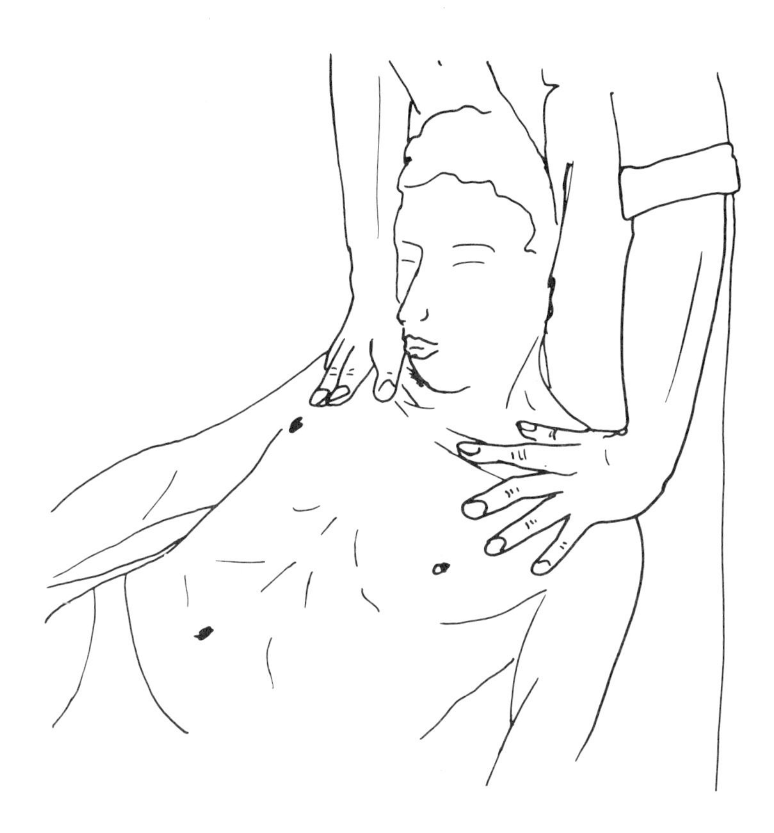

Illustration 5-20
Cervicopleural Test in the Supine Position

beginning, we tested these recesses by utilizing costal elasticity to mobilize them, but this approach ignored the sternochondral joints. We subsequently developed a more reliable test, as follows. Place the patient in the supine position, arms next to the body. Sit behind the head and place both your hands around the fourth sternochondrals. Apply pressure in the transverse plane, first toward the midline, then laterally. Firm but comfortable pressure is maintained during normal exhalation and inhalation. Next, ask the patient to inhale deeply. With a restriction the patient will feel intense and uncomfortable tension in the middle of the thorax. He may also experience a need to cough, or pain in the shoulders (similar to the pain felt during intense coughing, or attempts to defecate while constipated). With practice you will be able to perform this test using less pressure, and to tell whether the problem is unilateral or bilateral.

Costodiaphragmatic Recesses

For testing these structures, the areas of significance are the seventh costochondral joints, anterior parts of ribs 7 and 8, and posterior part of rib 11. The posterolateral part of the recess is easily accessible with the patient seated in front of you, legs hanging down, hands resting on the thighs. Place your hands on both sides of the thorax and ask the patient to exhale deeply. Press both thumbs against the posterior part of rib 11 and your index fingers against rib 8, pointing toward the seventh costochondral. When the patient inhales, compress the ribs medially and push them inferiorly. If there is a restriction of the costodiaphragmatic recesses, the patient will feel intense respiratory discomfort, the urge to cough, and tension in the thorax, sometimes extending as far as the supraclavicular fossae. These recesses are most likely to be affected by severe pleuropulmonary disorders. Because they are normally slack, they have considerable compensatory capacity, and are seldom affected by trauma due to car accidents, except when the lower ribs are fractured.

General Pleural Test

In this test, you create simultaneous tension of the costomediastinal and costodiaphragmatic recesses. Have the patient lie supine, legs straight, the arm on the side to be tested in external rotation and abduction, and the head sidebent and rotated toward the opposite side. Cross your arms and accentuate the sidebending rotation of the head with one hand in order to stretch the cervicopleural ligaments. Use the other hand to push the costodiaphragmatic recess inferomedially during inhalation (Illustration 5-21). Practice this test to learn what pleural mobility feels like. With a restriction, tension is too strong and the patient cannot inhale easily. Question him to learn the point in the breathing cycle when tension is most intense. With practice you will feel this without asking.

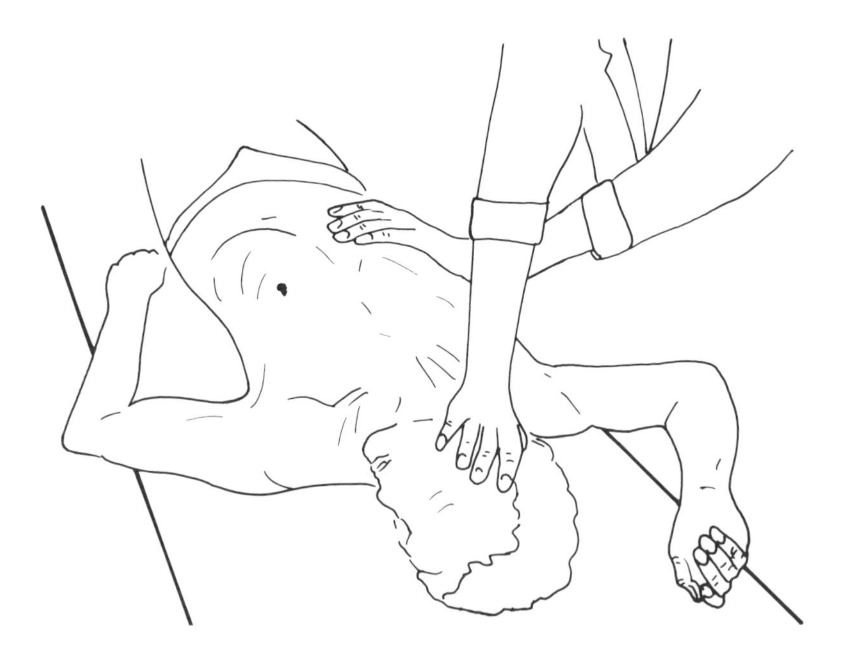

Illustration 5-21
General Pleural Test

Pericardium

We have less experience in this area than with pleural restrictions. With documented pericardial conditions, we have found that tensions are typically localized in the sternocostopericardial or vertebropericardial ligaments. The principal attachments of these ligaments are on the lower cervical vertebrae (usually C5-7), manubrium, and T4. The mobility test is easiest to perform in the supine position because of the increased tension on the ligaments. Again, have the patient lie supine, legs straight, arms alongside the body, head resting on your abdomen in right sidebending rotation. This puts the vertebropericardial ligaments under tension, as they are thicker and more resistant on the left side. Place one palm just below the manubrium and the other under the spinous process of T4. Increase the right sidebending rotation of the head while pulling T4 and the manubrium inferiorly and slightly to the left. You must repeat this test several times before reaching any conclusion. In the absence of restrictions, you cannot feel the pericardium. Interestingly, we have treated several patients with prior pericardial disorders in whom this stretching caused the heart rate to increase.

VISCERAL TESTS

Because of the presence of the ribcage, the intrathoracic viscera are relatively inaccessible, and difficult to test directly. It is usually more effective to test and manipulate their fasciae. Thus, this section is quite short. Motility of the lungs was covered in *Visceral Manipulation,* pp. 52-53.

Lungs

It is essentially impossible to test the lungs separately from the pleura. However, we have noticed that severe pleuropulmonary conditions often involve restrictions at specific lung fissures, and have had many opportunities to test these fissures in patients with chronic lung diseases. As other elements are involved in the tests described below, we like to refer to fissural regions, rather than fissures per se.

For the test of the *left horizontal fissural region,* place the patient in right lateral decubitus position, upper leg bent and lower leg extended for balance. Stand or sit behind the patient and place one palm on the posterior part of rib 5 on the left, close to the scapula, and the other palm on the anterior part of rib 6, close to the costochondral joint. During exhalation, let your hands go with the ribs as they move inferomedially (Illustration 5-22), and try to maintain this position during inhalation. If the patient feels discomfort or difficulty during inhalation, there may be a restriction of this region. Even if you have problems evaluating this test, this fissure should be treated in all patients with pleuropulmonary conditions, especially restrictions of the suspensory apparatus.

For the test of the *right horizontal fissural region,* the patient should be in left lateral decubitus position. Place the heel of one palm close to the lateral scapula between ribs 4 and 5, while the rest of that hand points in the direction of the third sternochondral and surrounds rib 4. Place your other hand on top of the first hand and push it inferolaterally during exhalation, as if focusing pressure on the third sternochondral joint. Maintain the pressure during inhalation and evaluate the patient's response as described above.

For the test of the *right oblique fissural region,* the patient is also in the left lateral decubitus position. Place one palm against the lateral scapula at the level of rib 5, the fingers of the hand pointing along the rib. Place the other palm beside it on rib 6, the fingers pointing in the direction of the sixth costochondral. Proceed as described above. We have tried this test in the prone position, but found that restrictions of the fissure are very difficult to distinguish from those of the costovertebral articulations. On the

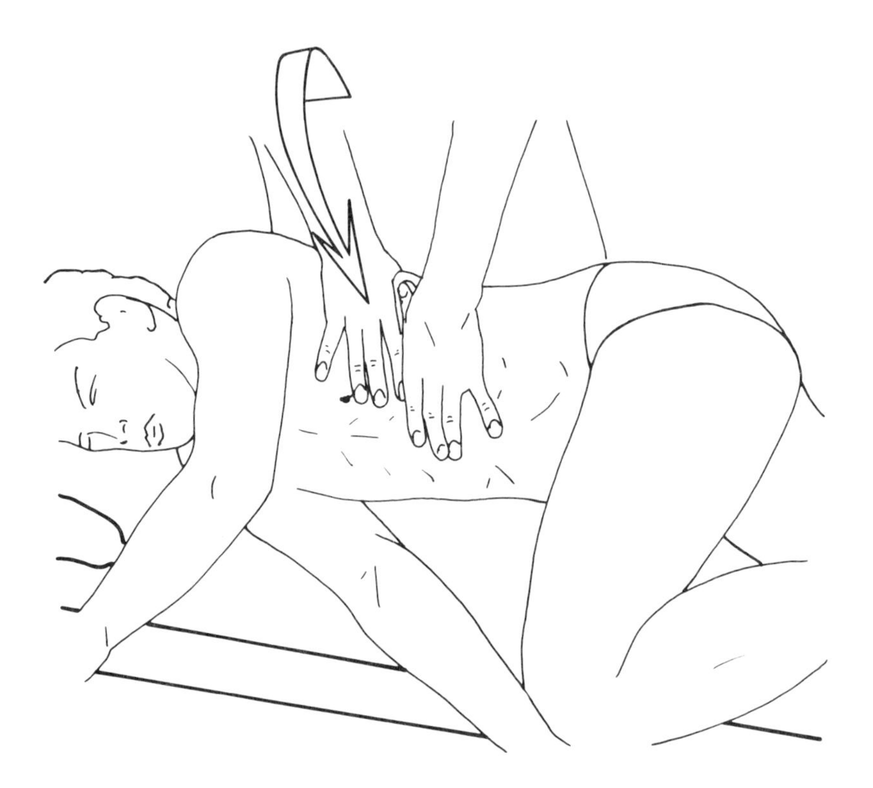

Illustration 5-22
Test of Left Horizontal Fissural Region

other hand, when the test is attempted in the supine position, a large part of the fissure is inaccessible.

These three tests are not specific for the respective fissures, because any mobilization of the thorax involves numerous elements. When we performed these tests on patients with sequelae from interlobar pleuritis, they experienced precisely the same pain as during the acute stage of the disease.

Other Organs

We frankly do not know of a practical mobility test for the *heart* as a whole. You can sometimes get useful information from the test for the superomedial part of the pericardium (see above), or from some stretching techniques applied along the orientation of the coronary arteries (see Chapter 6).

The *thymus*, likewise, does not have a specific test. This organ, like the spleen, is cause for concern if it is enlarged or palpable. Patients with such problems deserve a thorough work-up.

The *gastroesophageal junction* is often responsible for intrathoracic visceral problems, especially those due to gastroesophageal reflux. Refer to *Visceral Manipulation* (pp. 123-124) and *Visceral Manipulation II* (pp. 59-61) for appropriate tests.

Advice

Our general strategy for manual diagnosis is to proceed in the following order:

- general listening,
- local listening,
- osteoarticular testing,
- muscular and fascial testing,
- listening to the plexuses.

Perform the tests as rapidly and gently as possible because of the risk of creating restrictions during the testing process. If you are unsure of yourself, abandon the structure you are testing for another, and try again later.

Gentleness is important. The more pressure you exert during the test, the more you will feel your own fingers rather than the tissues of the patient.

Chapter Six: *Treatment*

Table of Contents

CHAPTER SIX

Treatment

General Principles

We remain firm believers in the Stillian concept of osteopathic treatment, based on the idea of freeing the affected structures. We interpret Still's statement, "The rule of the artery is supreme," as referring not only to the artery but also to its immediate anatomical environment. The thoracic inlet is the best example of the Stillian concept, as should become obvious in this chapter.

The osteopath uses his hands with great precision to exert corrective pressure on tissues which are in spasm, fixed, fibrosed, or have lost their natural distensibility. These dysfunctional tissues can produce a variety of symptoms and problems through irritation, disturbance, or compression of components of the neurovascular, visceral, or osteoarticular systems. One common example is inadequate arterial, venous, or lymphatic circulation. Another is local or regional nervous hyperexcitability leading to spasmodic restrictions of smooth muscle fibers. For example, an artery in spasm has its lumen reduced by vasoconstriction. General homeostasis is disturbed by such imbalances, which become progressively local, regional, and finally generalized. As discussed below, a simple restriction can lead to major pathology by the process of compensation/decompensation.

COMPENSATION/DECOMPENSATION

A healthy person is really one who has good compensatory abilities. All humans are affected by many forms of nervous stress which are essential for survival. They begin before birth and continue throughout life. The body retains a memory of all traumas it has experienced, regardless of type (infectious, vaccinatory, traumatic, psychological, metabolic, etc.) Environmental pollution is omnipresent and a permanent source of physiological stress. Apparent good health really represents efficient compensation (adaptation) to the environment, and most of us are close to the threshold of decompensation. Decompensation can take the form of a disproportionate reaction of the body to a stressor (physical, psychological, or other) which seems trivial. We have seen acute (even disabling) low back pain triggered by simply sneezing or bending to pick something off the floor.

We believe that it is overly simplistic to ascribe all low back pain to simple muscular tension or damaged intervertebral disks. Precipitating factors that we have run across include angina, acute colitis, genital infection, asthenia, and IUD insertion. Obviously, diseased disks do occur. But how does one explain the many cases of asymptomatic compressed disks, osteophytosis, cervical spondylosis, etc., that are revealed by modern imaging techniques?

The role of the osteopath is to improve overall equilibrium or homeostasis by delicately balancing the mechanical tensions of the body. Even if somatic dysfunctions represent only 20% of the total restrictions in a patient, osteopathic treatment can have a much farther-reaching effect by preventing decompensation. Therefore, we should train ourselves to recognize all tissue restrictions and treat them to the best of our ability.

RELEASE TECHNIQUES

Our therapeutic techniques may be directed toward joints, muscles, fasciae, ligaments, organs, or nervous plexuses. The thorax is a perfect example of the interdependence of the different structures and systems. This makes proper localization of your treatment both crucial and problematic. Release of an intercostal muscle, which is related to the pleura, can have a strong effect on the lung. As another example, a restriction in the acromioclavicular joint can affect the subclavian artery because of the resulting imbalance of reciprocal tensions in the thoracic inlet.

Joints

There are many ways to release joint restrictions. You can utilize traction on the periarticular soft tissues, the stretch reflexes of the small short muscles, or direct stretching of ligaments, muscular antagonists, or even intra-articular micro-adhesions. We are dubious of the efficacy of articular repositioning, except with dislocations (e.g., sternochondrals, coccyx) or when the bones have literally slid over one another (e.g., tibiotalar, tibiofibular). In our experience, such cases are fairly rare.

Muscles

Some small muscles, such as the rectus capitis or the intertransverse, can be released for a long time by our techniques. For example, manipulation of C2 has a longer-lasting effect than massage on these muscles. However, manipulation of the larger muscles gives a release that is both slight and short-term. We think of the large muscles, particularly quadratus lumborum, psoas, trapezius, and (sometimes) diaphragm, as the body's "overflow" or "wastebasket," since they collect the excess tension arising from the mechanical, metabolic, and psychological systems. A psoas in spasm is a symptomatic phenomenon, and its release is best left to those practitioners (physical therapists, deep tissue massage therapists, Rolfers, etc.) who are better trained for this kind of work.

Fasciae and Ligaments

These connective tissues are deceptively simple in appearance. Our colleagues Gabarel and Roques (1985) have published a detailed study on fascial techniques which inspires almost as many questions as it answers. Release of these tissues is accomplished by direct stretching in the directions indicated by testing. As with all soft tissues, the direction and speed of manipulation are crucial for optimal results. A stretching movement performed too slowly or in the wrong position may have little or no beneficial effect. We have been successful in using very gentle and quick manipulations to obtain relaxation in these tissues, although the mechanism for this is not clear. Certain fasciae, e.g., those around the mediastinum or heart, do not have specific tests; listening techniques are indispensable in these cases. Let the patient's body express its own tensions, and be honest about your own lack of knowledge. Sometimes listening may point to a tissue which you are not even familiar with. Try to release it, and later consult your anatomy books to identify it.

Generally the ligaments and tendons, like fasciae and muscles, contain Golgi receptors which are sensitive to stretching. In practice, manipulation has longer-lasting effects on fasciae than on tendons of long muscles. The ligaments of the pelvis are well supplied with contractile fibers, and we generally obtain good results from manipulation in the urogenital area. Contractile fibers are also present in the suspensory ligaments of the pleura, at the level of the hiatus (Juvara and Rouget's muscles), and in the suspensory system of the duodenojejunal junction (Treitz's muscle). Ligaments and fasciae are released by brief stretching, oriented in the direction of the fibers, sometimes using the recoil effect.

The fasciae are more affected by rapid trauma (e.g., motor vehicle accidents) than by slower forms of stress. Before attempting fascial release, you must have a precise and correct diagnosis. With car crashes, the thorax receives the majority of the force, and you need to know exactly which tissues (soft and hard) are affected. By using the appropriate tests and reaching a precise diagnosis, you will know what direction and force to use during treatment. Without a precise diagnosis you will end up pushing, pulling, and stretching the tissues in an aimless manner, to no avail.

Plexuses

Nervous plexuses of the thorax are networks of fibers arising mainly from the sympathetic and parasympathetic systems. In the past they were considered "peripheral brains." The important plexuses of the thorax are the celiac plexus, cardiac plexus, and stellate ganglion. During treatment, you will need to release them in this sequence and then coordinate them. Place your hand over the plexus and "listen." With a plexus which is overstimulated you will feel a fast, superficial motion, manifesting as a clockwise/counterclockwise rotation, a rocking motion, or even a motion directed interiorly from the surface. Go in the direction indicated by listening, slightly exaggerating what you feel, until your hand begins to slow down. If listening stops, your technique has been successful. It is essential, in the beginning, to **encourage** the motion you feel, and subsequently let it stop by itself. If you try to stop the motion, your technique will be ineffective.

Osteoarticular System

Treatment of the articulations generally consists of gentle, brief thrusts delivered with careful precision. Do not force the joint and **never** go beyond the limit of normal motion. We have found it best to carry out the technique using both hands simultaneously, crossing the arms to achieve a balanced position and facilitate a controlled, precise thrust. The force is slightly stronger than that for visceral recoil. It must be quick and applied in precisely the right direction. Obviously, you will need to use more force for larger, heavier patients, or stronger structures (e.g., coracoclavicular ligament). Accurate placement of the hands is of course extremely important. Recoil should not be applied to the same structure more than three times during one treatment session.

Joint manipulation is a technique that requires a great amount of skill and discipline. It cannot be learned merely by reading a book. For this reason, this section of our book should only be utilized by those readers with adequate training in this field.

In the remainder of this chapter, we will use two conventions: we will assume that the problem being treated is on the **right side,** and use the term "hand" to mean the **thenar or hypothenar eminence,** unless otherwise specified.

STERNOCLAVICULAR JOINT

As mentioned in Chapter 5, you should not try to correct a dislocation of this joint because of the risk of provoking chondritis. With restrictions or even dislocations of this joint, concentrate on relaxing the fascia. Treat both sides, even if only one seems to be restricted.

Posterior Sternoclavicular Ligament

For treatment of this ligament in the *supine position,* the patient lies down with hands on the abdomen and legs extended. Place one hand on the medial right clavicle and give a quick, light push posteriorly and superolaterally. You should feel the clavicle move posteriorly and then return. Repeating the technique twice is usually sufficient. You can also place the two hands side by side or use the other hand to move the right shoulder anteromedially.

For treatment in the *seated position,* the patient sits facing away from you, legs hanging down. Place your right foot on the table and lay the patient's arm on your right thigh. Surround the right shoulder with your hand and push it anteromedially, while using the left hand to bring the medial right clavicle posteriorly and slightly laterally.

Anterior Sternoclavicular Ligament

Supine position: Exert pressure with your left palm on the lateral clavicle (near the acromioclavicular joint), and with your right palm or fingers on the superior edge of the medial clavicle (as deeply as possible). Push laterally and slightly anteriorly with the right hand, and inferolaterally with the left. In some cases you can actually lift the clavicle by focusing the movement on its medial end. Alternatively, cross your hands in such a way that (assuming that the problem is on the right) the heel of your right hand is on the sternum next to the left sternoclavicular, and the heel of your left hand is on the lateral right clavicle. Push the left hand posterolaterally, which will bring the medial clavicle anteriorly. The right palm increases this effect by pushing the left side of the sternum posterolaterally (Illustration 6-1). This technique is useful when the subclavian or brachiocephalic vessels are being compressed.

Seated position: The patient faces away from you, his left arm resting on your knee. Place the palm of your hand in the right supraclavicular fossa. Your index finger presses on the medial clavicle, while the thumb presses against the posterior angle of rib 1 and

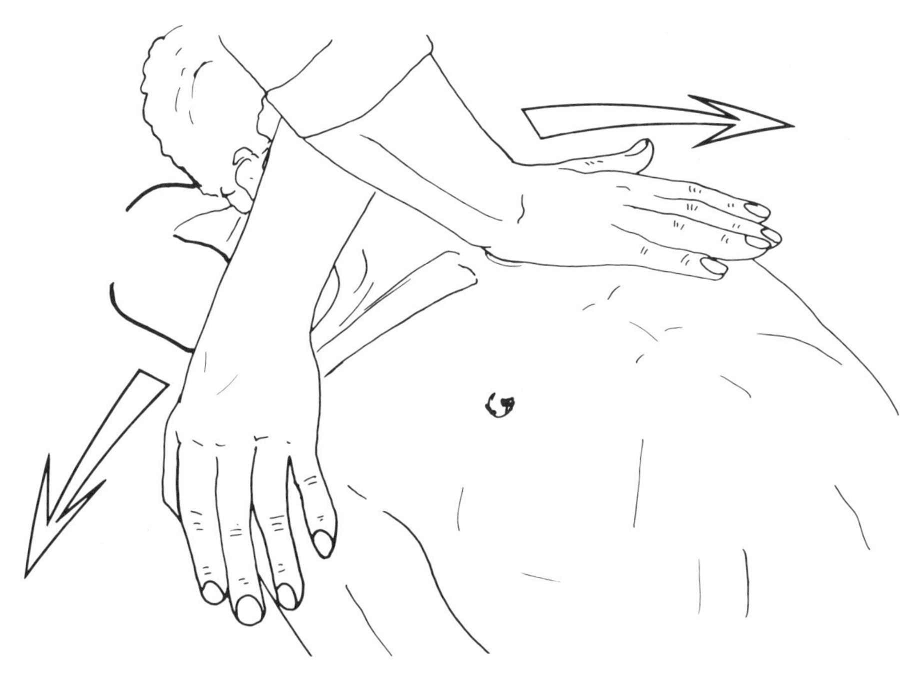

Illustration 6-1
Manipulation of the Anterior Sternoclavicular Ligament: Supine Position

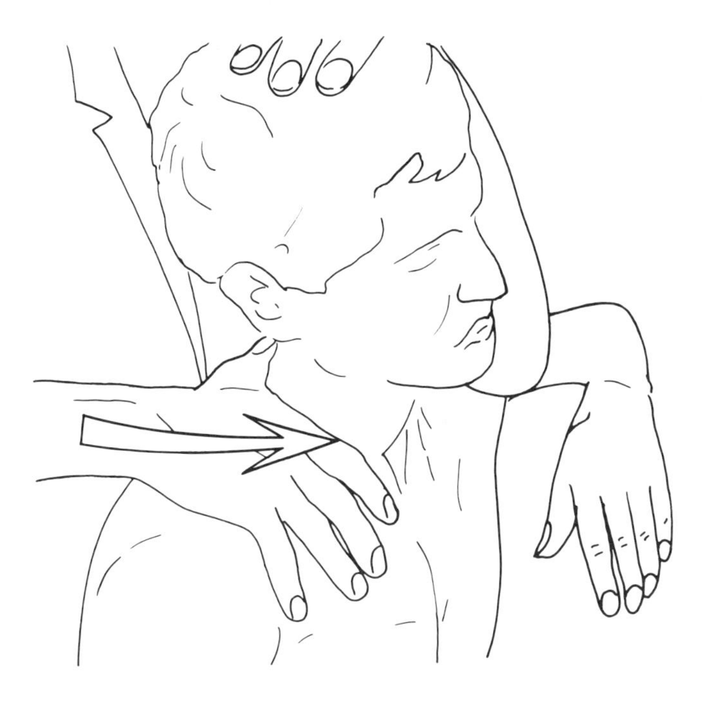

Illustration 6-2
Manipulation of the Anterior Sternoclavicular Ligament: Seated Position

the first costovertebral joint. Place the other hand on the left parietal bone, with your elbow resting on the patient's shoulder (Illustration 6-2). The "clavicular" hand pushes anteroinferiorly and toward the left side, while the hand on the skull sidebends the cervical spine toward the right. The entire thorax moves as you push on the clavicle, and you have a sense of utilizing the elasticity of the whole body. The thrust is given when tension is at its peak; the force comes only from the clavicular hand.

Interclavicular Ligament

Use this technique after you have treated the sternoclavicular ligaments. Place both hands in the suprasternal fossa, pressing against the medial sides of the sternoclavicular joints. The thrust is applied inferolaterally and very slightly anteriorly, usually with recoil.

ACROMIOCLAVICULAR JOINT

Again, do not try to push the clavicle back into place if there is a dislocation. Your job is to release the affected tissues so as to improve their elasticity. With a dislocation, certain fibers will be torn; these cannot be helped by osteopathic treatment, but the surrounding tissues can. After manipulation, the dislocation still exists but the patient suffers less.

Supine position: Stand on the right side near the patient's head. Cross your arms and place your left and right hypothenar eminences against the medial acromion and middle clavicle, respectively. Push posterolaterally with the left hand while the right moves the clavicle superomedially.

Seated position: The patient faces away from you. The technique is similar to that for the supine position, except that the pressure on the acromion is more inferior than posterior. Thoracic elasticity can be utilized in this position to increase the efficacy of manipulation.

CORACOCLAVICULAR LIGAMENTS

The trapezoid and conoid ligaments are often involved in restrictions of the subclavius muscle, which typically have an adverse effect on surrounding vascular circulation. The best strategy is to treat the subclavius first, and then the coracoclavicular ligaments. The patient should be in supine position.

Trapezoid ligament: Cross your hands and place one hand so as to stabilize the medial coracoid. Place the other hand on the medial acromioclavicular joint and push in a superolateral direction.

Conoid ligament: Similar technique as above, except that you place the second hand on the lateral third of the anterior edge of the clavicle, and press posterosuperiorly and medially (Illustration 6-3).

Acromiocoracoid ligament: This ligament does not have such a specific role as the other two. However, it may develop micro-adhesions following major trauma to the shoulder, and manipulation can restore its elasticity. With your arms crossed, place one hand against the acromion and the other against the coracoid. Push your hands in opposite directions: superolaterally and inferomedially, respectively.

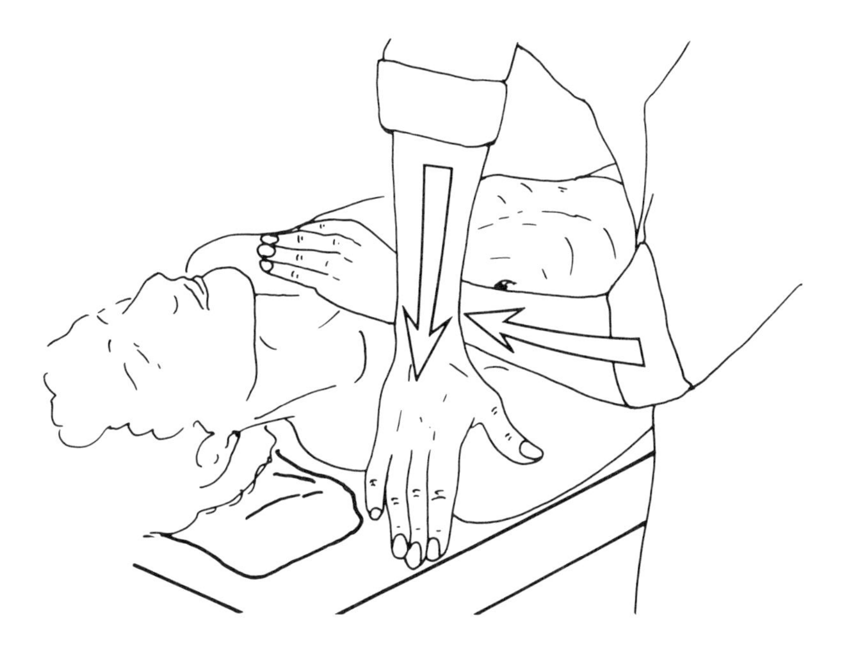

Illustration 6-3
Manipulation of the Conoid Ligament

GENERAL CLAVICULAR RELEASE

This technique is appropriate after direct trauma to the shoulder, especially due to seat belt impact. The sternoclavicular and acromioclavicular ligaments are stretched, and the elasticity of the clavicle itself is utilized. The patient should be in supine position. To use *longitudinal compression,* place one hand against the clavicular part of the acromioclavicular joint and the other on the medial clavicle. Push the hands towards each other and, when maximal tension is reached, let them go (Illustration 6-4). This is a good recoil technique. To use *longitudinal decompression,* the patient is in the same position but your arms are crossed and push away from each other. When you feel the maximum of tension, release the pressure.

STERNUM

This heavy bone is the most anterior structure of the thorax and generally the first to be affected by physical trauma. We consider it to be the "receptacle" of all thoracic trauma. Despite its prominence and vulnerability, it has been curiously neglected by manual medicine. We hope that this book will begin to remedy this situation.

Sternomanubrial Joint

Restriction of this joint is always associated with that of the second sternochondral. Treatment can be done by compression or decompression. We use these techniques for sequelae of thoracic trauma or following pleuropericardial problems. The patient lies supine with arms alongside the body. Stand to the side and press one hand against the

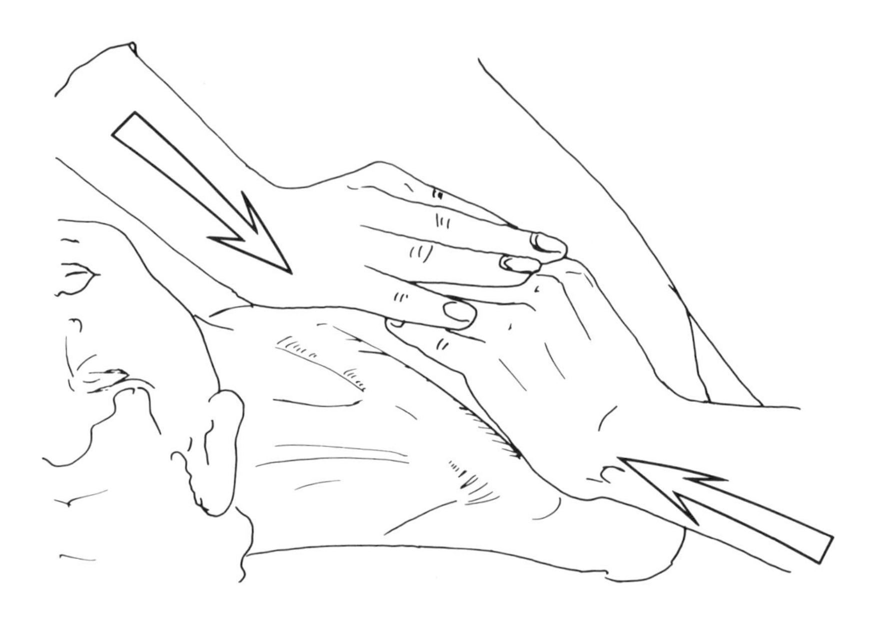

Illustration 6-4
General Clavicular Release with Longitudinal Compression

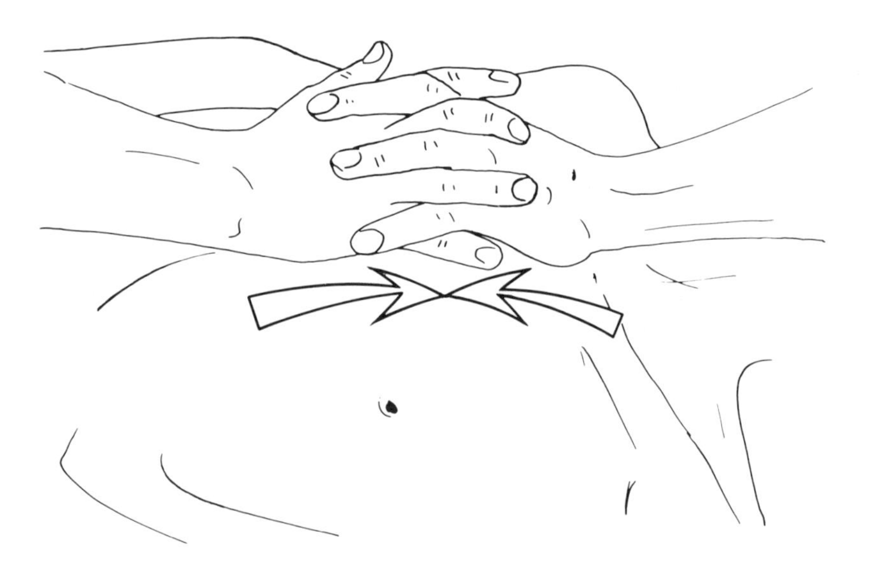

Illustration 6-5
Manipulation of the Sternomanubrial Joint with Longitudinal Compression

suprasternal fossa, just touching the superior border of the manubrium. Place the other hand just inferior to the sternal angle. Compression means pushing your hands together as if trying to make this angle more acute. At maximal tension, quickly release the pressure (Illustration 6-5). For decompression, the hands are crossed and carry out the opposite movement, stretching the sternum longitudinally. This can also be done as a recoil technique if the stretch is released quickly. These techniques release longitudinal tensions of the bony fibers as well as some of the anteroposterior tensions of the mediastinum.

Induction by Sternal Lifting

The patient lies supine with hands on the abdomen. Stand to the side and place one index finger against the jugular notch (underneath it if possible) and the other index finger against or under (depending on the patient) the xiphoid process. Use both fingers to compress the sternum by lifting it very slightly. You should then feel the sternum move very slightly in one direction or another. We call this the direction of listening. As in all induction techniques, you follow this direction, and then let the structure come back. Remember to slightly encourage the direction in which the motion is easiest. Repeat this several times until there is a release and you feel no further motion.

Sternal lifting is carried out following all direct techniques in order to balance the sternothoracic reciprocal tensions. It is also the best treatment for the xiphoid process, apart from the rare cases when true dislocation requires a direct lateral technique. Restrictions of the xiphoid produce few symptoms, unless there is a hiatal hernia or imbalance of hiatal myofascial tensions. Our observations suggest that a xiphoidal restriction can actually contribute to the development of a hiatal hernia by creating imbalances of tissues in this area.

Sternovertebral Technique

The patient is supine with arms alongside the body. Hold his head against your abdomen and flex the cervical spine. Place one hand on the sternum, palm against the sternal angle. The other hand is placed against the thoracic spine, with the heel at T4. Push the sternal hand inferiorly and slightly posteriorly, and the other hand superiorly (Illustration 6-6). At maximal tension, release the hands with recoil. Repeat this two or three times, then reverse the direction of the two hands; i.e., push the sternal hand superiorly and the other hand inferiorly and release, again using recoil. This technique is useful for sequelae of thoracic trauma (e.g., restrictions of the thoracic spine), or following pleurocardiopulmonary conditions.

Sternochondral Joints

Unlike many practitioners, we pay close attention to these articulations, which are often affected by such traumas as falls on the hands or seat belt impact. Restrictions here can lead to precordial pain, tachycardia, dyspnea with exertion, recurring thoracic vertebral restrictions, or feelings of uneasiness or general thoracic discomfort which are increased in the lateral decubitus and prone positions. During treatment, the patient should be supine, hands on the abdomen. Most sternochondral restrictions are either anterior or posterior. These restrictions are usually actual subluxations.

For *anterior subluxations,* stand to one side with one hand on the chondral portion of the joint, against the sternum, while the other hand lifts the right arm by the wrist. First move your hands away from each other to focus the tension on the correct sternochondral joint. This step is very important and can only be performed by varying the position of the arm. Then press posteriorly and slightly laterally with the sternal hand

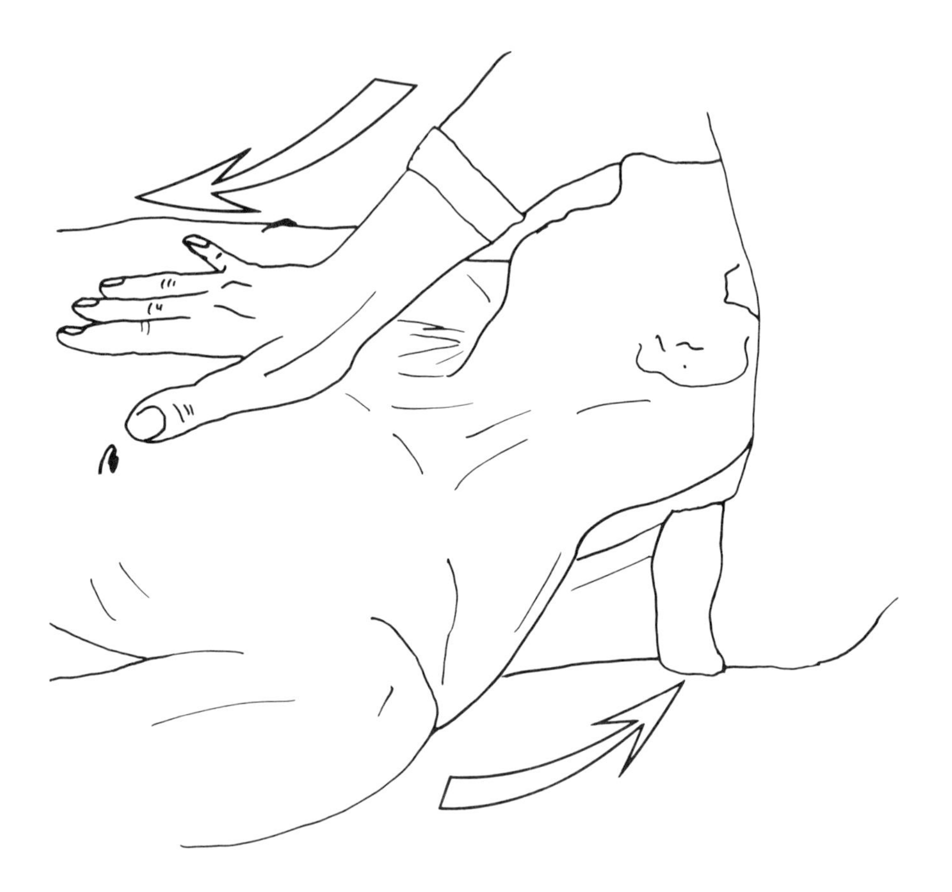

Illustration 6-6
Sternovertebral Technique

while further lifting the right arm in order to maximize the tension. At the point of maximal tension, give a light thrust with the sternal hand in the same direction you are already pressing (Illustration 6-7). You will sometimes hear the characteristic noise like that which accompanies vertebral adjustments. The thrust must be **very gentle.** Too much force can cause chondritis or a restriction of the corresponding costochondral joint. You can also perform induction starting at the point of maximal tension: using both hands in unison, follow the motion of the tissues until it stops.

For *posterior subluxation,* two methods are possible. The first is similar to that described above, except that the thoracic hand is placed on the sternal portion of the joint. Be sure that there is a balance between the traction on the arm and pressure on the chest before you thrust.

The second method utilizes respiration. The patient is supine and you are standing next to his head. With your hands crossed put one hand against the chondral portion of the joint, while stabilizing the sternal portion with the other hand. Ask the patient to breathe in and out deeply several times. During exhalation, push the sternum posteriorly and the chondral part slightly laterally. Relax the pressure just when the patient starts to inhale. All the thoracic forces will be concentrated on the pressure of your hand,

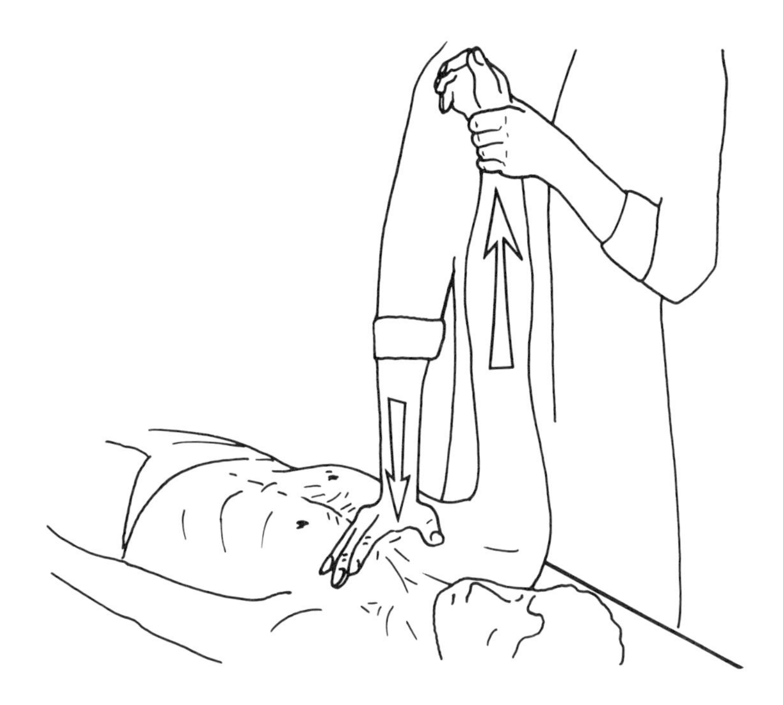

Illustration 6-7
Sternochondral Manipulation: Anterior Subluxation

freeing the chondral part anteriorly. Repeat this two or three times. Such recoil techniques with respiratory assistance are very effective. They should be distinguished from recoil performed without respiratory assistance, which is often applied to the joints of the arms and legs.

Sometimes the sternochondral joint is irritated and extremely painful. This may occur due to an inflammatory process or because someone has pushed on it too hard or too often. In these cases do not touch that articulation; rather treat the opposite sternochondral joint. This often helps considerably. We believe this effect is due to the crossing over of fibers between the two sides.

Costochondral Joints

The technique here is similar to that for the sternochondrals, except that your hand is on the rib instead of the sternum. For an anterior subluxation, use one hand to push posteriorly and slightly laterally on the rib, and the other to lift the left arm by the wrist. Posterior subluxations are treated with the thoracic hand on the cartilage. Your pressure should be less than in the sternochondral technique because the costochondral cartilage is very fragile. Although costochondral restrictions are often corrected by sternochondral release, you must systematically check and treat both areas. These joints are in perpetual movement with respiration, which explains their vulnerability to restrictions. The first costochondral is manipulated with the subclavius muscle, as described in the next section.

Muscular System

SUBCLAVIUS

Although this muscle is neglected by many manual therapists, restrictions here can affect the subclavian vascular system. The subclavius muscle, the costoclavicular ligament, and the first costochondral joint should be treated together, with the goal of separating the clavicle from rib 1 and loosening the associated muscles and fasciae. These techniques are useful after trauma to the shoulder or thorax, or falls onto the hands or elbows. They can also be used for upper respiratory problems, particularly those that occur after tuberculosis or pleuritis.

For treatment in the *supine position,* the patient lies with arms and legs stretched out. Stand on the right side and use one hand to hold the wrist or shoulder. Place the thumb of the other hand between the clavicle and rib 1, as close as possible to their sternal articulations. Move the right shoulder anteromedially until you feel tension under your thumb. At maximal tension, quickly but gently push rib 1 posterolaterally. During the manipulation you can simultaneously put the arm under brief traction. One or two

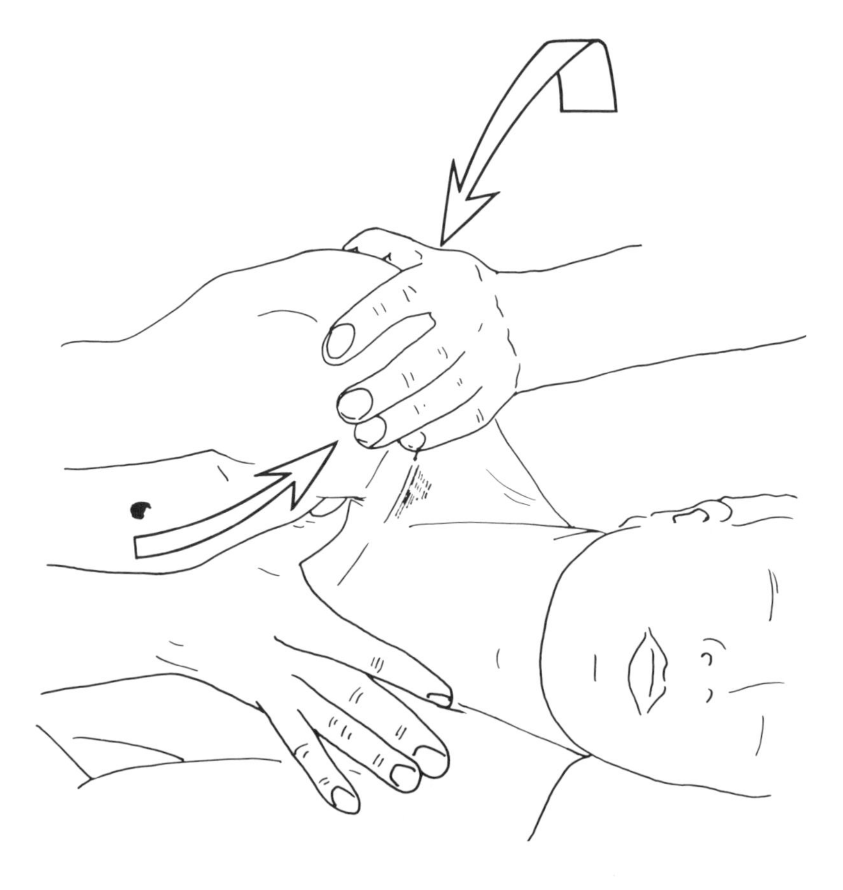

Illustration 6-8
Manipulation of the Subclavius Muscle: Lateral Decubitus Position

repetitions of this technique are usually sufficient. Alternatively, cross your arms and place one hand against the medial clavicle and the other on ribs 1 and 2. The clavicular hand pushes superolaterally while the costal hand pushes quickly inferomedially.

For treatment in the *lateral decubitus position,* the patient lies on his left side. Place one palm on the sternum with the thumb between the medial clavicle and rib 1, the other palm on the posterior shoulder. Push posterolaterally with the thumb while moving the shoulder anteromedially (Illustration 6-8). At maximal tension, give a quick, gentle thrust.

For treatment in the *seated position,* stand behind the patient and reach around so that your thumb (or thenar eminence) is between the medial part of rib 1 and the clavicle. Hold the right shoulder with the other hand. Move the shoulder anteromedially and press your thumb posterolaterally. Again, give a quick, gentle thrust at maximal tension. Alternatively, put your foot on the table and let the patient's right arm rest on your thigh. This position allows you to move the patient's shoulder using your leg. To further stretch the subclavius muscle, lift up the shoulder before bringing it anteromedially.

TRANSVERSUS THORACIS

This muscle is treated in combination with the sternum and intercostal muscles; there is no specific technique. It is a good idea to stretch the transversus thoracis with significant thoracic restrictions or following a pleural disorder. Put the patient in supine position, arms and legs stretched out. Stand on the right side and cross your arms. Place one hand below the manubrium (the fibers of this muscle insert only on the inferior third of the sternum), and the other on the middle ribs, near the costochondral joints. Press

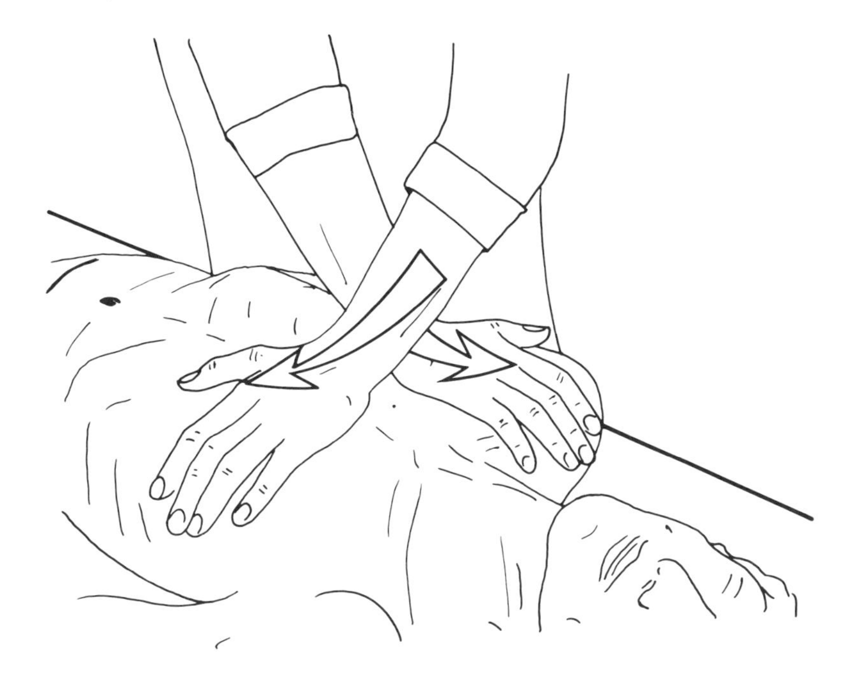

Illustration 6-9
Sternocostal Manipulation Focusing on the Transversus Thoracis Muscle

the sternal hand posterosuperiorly, and use the costal hand to move the ribs in an inferolateral direction (Illustration 6-9). Repeat on the other side. Sometimes we have found this technique to release restrictions of which we were not even aware!

EXTERNAL INTERCOSTALS

For convenience, we will divide these muscles into anterolateral and posterior portions. For treatment of the anterolateral portion in the *supine position,* stand on the patient's left side and cross your arms. Place one hand on the sternum, and the other against the lower edge of the rib above the affected muscle. As the patient exhales, maintain the position of the rib by pushing superolaterally, while pushing the sternum posteroinferiorly. Best results are obtained by holding this stretch during exhalation because costal elasticity is relatively increased during this phase of respiration. For the alternative method in the *lateral decubitus position,* stand behind the patient, hold the left arm with one hand, and place the palm of the other hand on the upper edge of the rib below the affected muscle. Move the arm posterosuperiorly until you feel tension with the costal hand (Illustration 6-10). As with the sternochondral techniques, at maximal tension you should gently and quickly thrust (or stretch) two to three times.

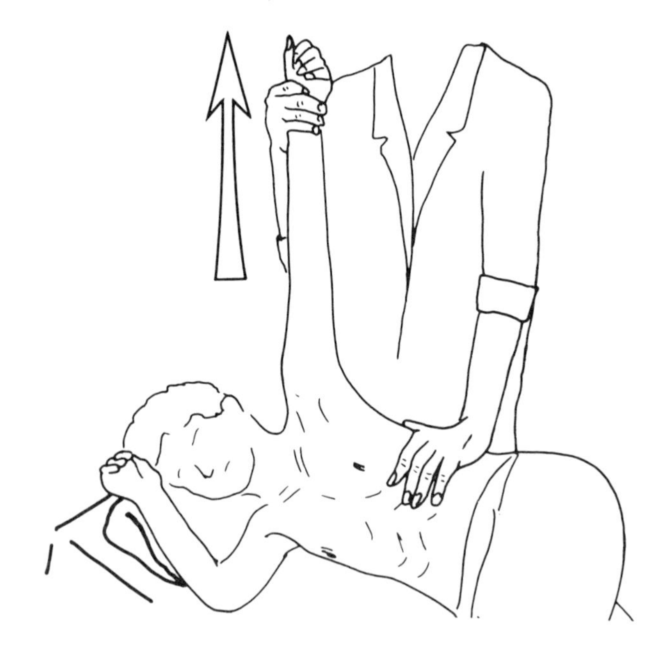

Illustration 6-10
Manipulation of the External Intercostal Muscles: Lateral Decubitus Position

For treatment of the *posterior portion* of the external intercostals, put the patient in prone position, arms at the sides, head rotated to the left. Cross your arms and place one hand on the lateral part of the posterior angle of the rib above the affected muscle. Place your other hand on the superior edge of the rib below the muscle, just medial to the angle. At maximal tension (which will be at the end of exhalation) push your hands in opposite directions, quickly and gently.

These techniques can be adapted for recoil with respiratory assistance (see "Sternochondral joints" above). Have the patient breathe deeply. Simply maintain muscular/ligamentous tension at the end of exhalation and instantly release it at the beginning of inhalation. The patient may report some pain in the shoulder or supraclavicular fossa, and have a slight irritable cough. These are the same symptoms found in pleural stretching, and indicate that you have effectively treated the pleural attachments.

INTERNAL INTERCOSTALS

The techniques are similar to those for the external intercostals, but the direction of force is changed. For example, to treat the anterior portion, cross your arms, place one hand on the upper edge of the rib below the affected muscle, and the other against the lateral edge of the sternum. Push the costal hand posterolaterally and inferiorly, and the sternal hand superomedially. You can try putting pressure on the adjacent rib instead of the sternum, but this is more difficult; often the intercostal space is too narrow.

LEVATORES COSTARUM

These muscles can be tight due to trauma or pleural problems. Usually when trauma is the cause the area of restriction is relatively localized (1-4 ribs are involved); when it is due to a pleural problem the restrictions are more diffuse. Treating the posterior aspect of the ribs is extremely important. If you only treat the anterior aspects the restrictions will recur within a couple of weeks.

The patient is prone, arms hanging over the edge of the table, head rotated to the left. Place one hand between the spinous and transverse processes of the affected vertebra and the other on the posterior angle of the adjacent inferior rib (or, for the four lower vertebrae, the rib two segments below). The vertebral hand stabilizes the vertebra or even pushes it slightly in a superomedial direction, while the costal hand pushes anterolaterally and inferiorly. At maximal tension (usually at the very end of exhalation), give a quick gentle thrust. Recoil with respiratory assistance can also be used.

DIAPHRAGM

We do not have any specific treatments for the diaphragm. We work indirectly through organs (e.g., liver, colon), muscles (e.g., intercostals), or bones (ribs, vertebrae). As mentioned in Chapter 5, we doubt the existence of primary restrictions of the diaphragm. If an apparent restriction is due to emotional, digestive, or osteoarticular factors, you must treat the primary cause. With emotional causes, treatment of the plexuses or the phrenic nerve (described later in this chapter) may be helpful. Techniques for various digestive disorders are described in our previous books.

Fascial System

MIDDLE CERVICAL APONEUROSIS

As explained in Chapters 2 and 5, this structure plays a central role in thoracic function. It is affected by all trauma to the cervical spine or thorax, as well as by all cardiac or pleuropulmonary disorders. Due to its vascular connections, it is often involved in circulatory problems of the cervicothoracic junction.

For treatment in the *supine position,* the patient's arms and legs are extended and his head rests on your abdomen. Place one hand with the thumb in the right supraclavicular fossa against rib 1, toward the scalene tubercle, and the heel on the superior edge of the scapula. To position the thumb correctly, sidebend the neck to the right. Your other hand can press between rib 1 and the clavicle to stretch the subclavius muscle, hold the cervical spine, or even stabilize the left shoulder (Illustration 6-11).

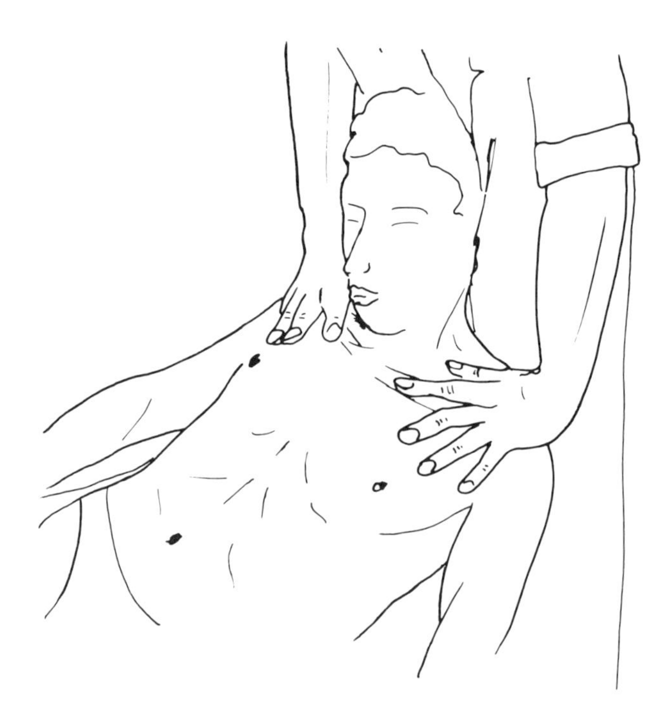

Illustration 6-11
Manipulation of the Middle Cervical Aponeurosis: Supine Position

Use your abdomen to sidebend the cervical spine to the left until you feel fascial tension with the thumb and palm of the treating hand. The thumb is meanwhile searching for areas which are more tense in order to "fine-tune" their stretching. By varying the degree of forward bending of the cervical spine, you can focus the stretching on the anterior or posterolateral part of the aponeurosis. This technique should be comfortable for both you and the patient. Be sure the pressure exerted by your thumb is not too great.

We have not found direct techniques with stabilization of the hyoid bone to be effective. However, induction techniques for this aponeurosis do seem to be more effective when one hand is placed over the hyoid and the other against the medial clavicle and rib 1. Induction, as usual, consists of going in the direction of listening and returning repeatedly until the motion stops.

For treatment of the middle cervical aponeurosis in the *seated position,* the patient's back is against you, your foot on the table, and his left arm resting on your thigh. Place your right hand with the index finger along the right clavicle with the tip on the sternoclavicular joint, and the thumb near the superior edge of the scapula. Place the left hand on the patient's head, your elbow resting on the left shoulder. The treating hand pushes the clavicle anteroinferiorly and medially, while the other hand sidebends and rotates the neck slightly to the left. This is shown for a restriction on the left in Illustration 6-12. At maximal tension, give a quick gentle thrust. Using your leg, you can vary the position of the thorax to increase fascial tension. This technique requires good coordination and synchronization of your whole body, and can be very effective.

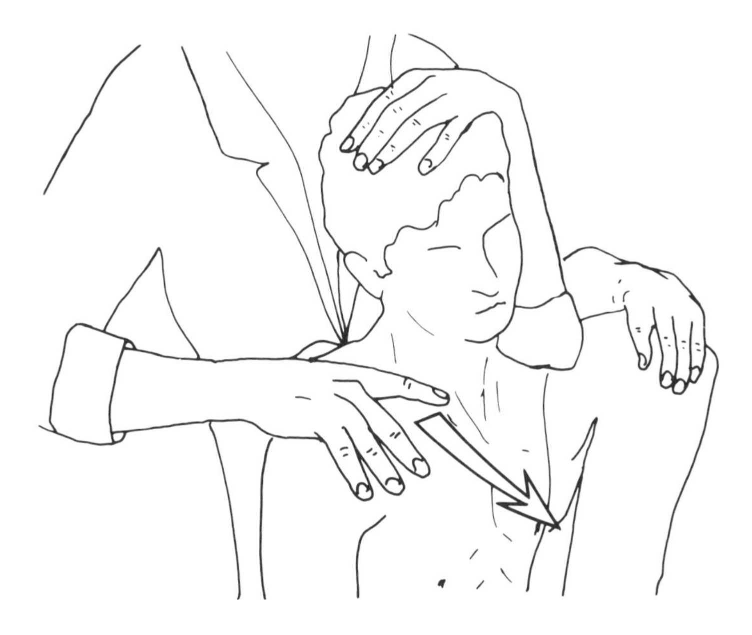

Illustration 6-12
Manipulation of the Middle Cervical Aponeurosis: Seated Position

Always remember to release the subclavius muscle and conoid and trapezoid ligaments before treating a middle cervical aponeurosis. If these associated structures remain restricted, you will not be able to release the aponeurosis.

CLAVIPECTORAL FASCIA

This fascia is typically affected by falls onto the shoulder or lateral thorax. Treatment here is especially helpful for pain which radiates downward from the clavicles.

For treatment in the *supine position,* put the patient's right arm into external rotation and abduction (to fix part of the brachial aponeurosis), and rest his head against your abdomen. Cross your arms, place both hands on the coracoid processes, and push them posterolaterally and slightly inferiorly. Use your abdomen to sidebend the neck to the left. At maximal tension, give a thrust with the hand on the right (Illustration 6-13). The bending of the neck stretches the middle cervical aponeurosis, which inserts along with the clavipectoral onto the aponeurosis of the subclavius muscle.

For treatment in the *seated position,* the patient's back is against you, his left arm resting on your thigh, and your foot on the table. Place one palm (usually the left) against the right coracoid process. Use the other hand to hold the head and sidebend the neck

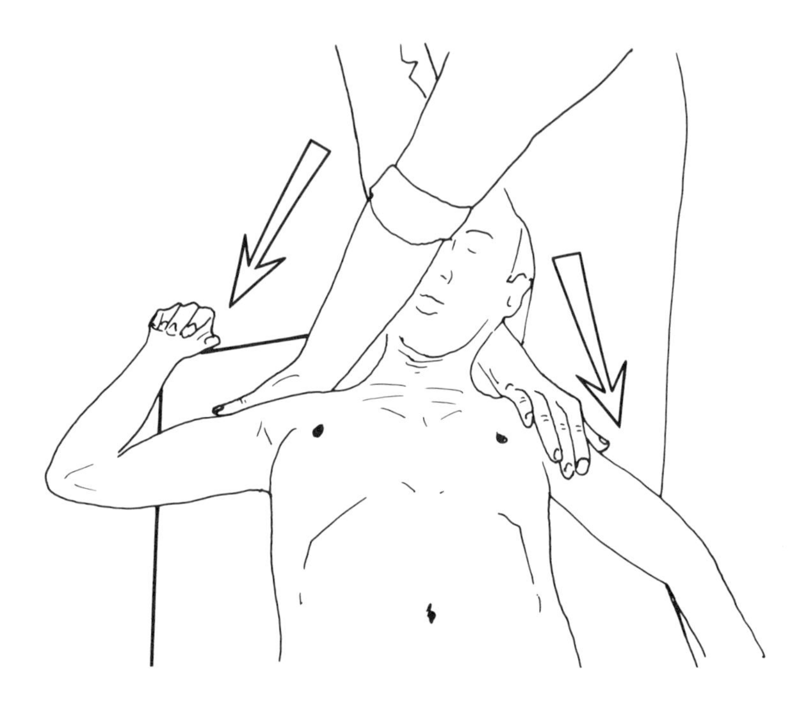

Illustration 6-13
Manipulation of the Clavipectoral Fascia: Supine Position

so that maximal tension is focused on the middle cervical aponeurosis. Give a quick gentle thrust, in an inferolateral direction, to the coracoid process.

Release of the axillary fossa is performed in cases of very painful cervicobrachial neuralgia. The patient may be seated with the practitioner behind him, or supine with the practitioner to the side. The patient's elbow is on your thigh. Place one hand on the right shoulder and use the fingers of the other hand to probe the axillary fossa in search of fascial tensions. These are then released by plucking the fibers like guitar strings. It goes without saying that you may find certain surprises anytime you put your hand in someone's axillary fossa. You can treat cervicobrachial neuralgia in the same way, using the nerves of the brachial plexus. This "guitar string" technique must be done gently so as to avoid creating uncomfortable and long-lasting paresthesias.

PLEURA

Some practitioners concentrate on loosening the middle and lower parts of the pleura, and ignore the superior attachments. However, these are equally important.

Cervicopleural Suspensory Apparatus

In the *seated position,* the myofascial tensions and intrathoracic pressures are normal and easier to work with. The patient has his back against you, and his left arm resting on your thigh. Place the thumb or index finger of one hand deeply behind the clavicle, against the scalene tubercle, with the palm oriented along the clavicle. Use the other hand to rotate and sidebend the patient's head to the left, so as to put the cervicopleural fibers under tension. The treating hand then performs the "guitar string" technique on the cervicopleural ligaments. Next, ask the patient to breathe deeply. During inhalation, push rib 1 inferolaterally and slightly posteriorly, and simultaneously rotate and sidebend the cervical spine to the left. Repeat this until the tension is released. Usually 4-5 repetitions are enough. This is a fairly strong stretching technique. Always begin very gently and gradually, and stop if the patient feels pain in the chest, which may happen if you irritate the vagus nerve or one of the vertebrae. This technique can also be adapted for recoil with respiratory assistance. When the suspensory apparatus is at maximal tension, ask the patient to exhale deeply. Just before inhalation, quickly release the pressure on the clavicle and ribs. You should see the thorax moving upward like a spring.

For treatment of the cervicopleural suspensory apparatus in the *supine position*, the patient rests his hands on his abdomen, and his head on your abdomen. Place the thumb of your right hand on rib 1 near the scalene tubercle, and the palm against the clavicle. Place your left hand on the left clavicle for counter-pressure. Use your abdomen to forward bend the cervical spine, and then sidebend it to the left. At the same time, use your right hand to push the clavicle and rib 1 posterolaterally and inferiorly, and give a thrust at maximal tension. You can also use recoil with respiratory assistance. These techniques should be performed bilaterally in order to balance the reciprocal upper pleural pressures, which are considerable.

If the patient feels a tingling of the fingers during one of these techniques you have placed your fingers too posteriorly, laterally, and superiorly. If you persist in attempting to treat them when this happens you can cause a temporary cervicobrachial neuralgia. This can last for two to three weeks.

Middle Pleura

The costomediastinal recesses and parietal pleura of the middle thorax are treated with the patient supine, head resting on your abdomen. Cross your arms and press the palm of one hand against ribs 3 through 5, lateral to the costochondral joints, and the other against the middle part of the sternum. At the end of exhalation, move the costal hand posterolaterally and inferiorly, and the sternal hand laterally and slightly superiorly, following the direction of the opposite ribs. Maintain the pressure and use recoil with respiratory assistance.

General Manipulation of the Pleura

We have not been convinced of the efficacy of treating the costomediastinal recesses by themselves. We therefore prefer to integrate their treatment with the general treatment of the pleura, as described here. For the treatment in the *supine position*, the patient's hands are alongside the body, and his legs bent to the left and resting on the table. His head is also sidebent and rotated to the left. With your arms crossed, place one hand on the head to increase the sidebending rotation of the cervical column, and the other on the costodiaphragmatic recess, over the seventh costochondral joint. Push the costal hand inferolaterally (Illustration 6-14). At maximal tension (during inhalation), quickly release the pressure of both hands. This is recoil with respiratory assistance. You can also continue the stretching motion of the hands as the patient exhales slowly and deeply. An alternative method in this position also utilizes recoil with respiratory assistance. Keep

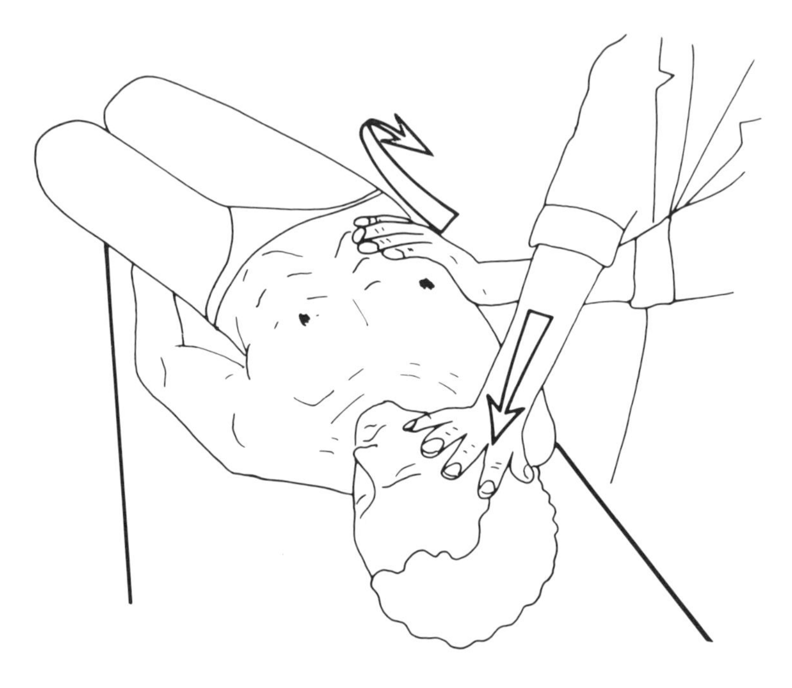

Illustration 6-14
General Manipulation of the Pleura: Supine Position

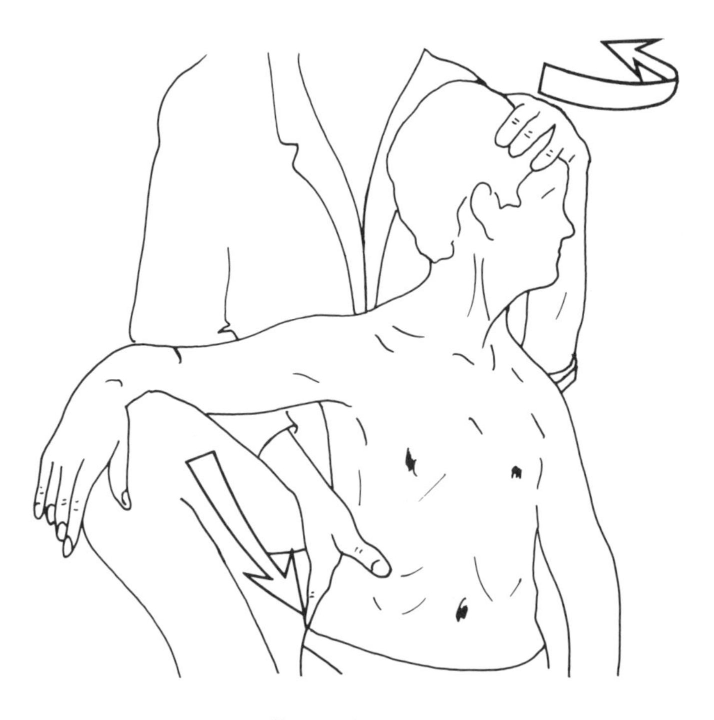

Illustration 6-15
General Manipulation of the Pleura: Seated Position

your arms uncrossed and place the second hand over the right clavicle and rib 1 instead of on the head. As the patient exhales slowly and deeply, move your hands toward each other within the limits allowed by the compression; this will literally compress the thorax. Release the pressure of both hands just at the beginning of a quick, deep inhalation. This technique will relax the hemithorax and corresponding pleura.

For general manipulation of the pleura in the *seated position,* the patient's back is against you, his right arm resting on your thigh. Use your right hand to hold the lateral parts of ribs 9 through 11, while your left hand sidebends and rotates the head to the left. Your right hand, assisted by the support of your leg, pushes the ribs inferomedially (Illustration 6-15). When you feel maximal tension, ask the patient to exhale deeply and then "freeze" so that you can increase the pressure a little more. Maintain this pressure (which keeps the pleura in a position of exhalation) while the patient inhales; as the diaphragm moves downward it will stretch the pleura. An alternative direct stretching technique involves changing the direction of the superior pressure. The patient puts his right hand behind his head. Your second hand moves the elbow posterosuperiorly and medially, while your costal hand pushes anteroinferiorly and medially. The rest of the technique is as described above.

PERICARDIUM AND MEDIASTINUM

There are no specific techniques for these fasciae. We cannot see how stretching of the pericardium could be separated from stretching of the mediastinum. The techniques described above for the sternum, using either the supine or seated position, work well for these structures. In these cases we prefer to use recoil with respiratory assistance.

Viscera

LUNGS

The following techniques are obviously not very specific, since they affect many other structures besides the lung fissures. Nevertheless, they have been shown to be effective. They are useful with patients with sequelae of serious pulmonary problems, or complaints of pain in the cervical or thoracic spine.

For treatment of the *left horizontal fissural region,* put the patient in right lateral decubitus position. Place your right hand on rib 5 near the scapula, and the left on the anterior part of rib 6 near its costochondral joint. While the patient exhales slowly and deeply, push your palms anteroinferiorly and medially, focusing the movement toward the sixth sternochondral joint. Maintain this pressure while the patient inhales deeply (Illustration 6-16). Repeat until you feel a release. Again, the diaphragm is used to provide the force for stretching. To use recoil with respiratory assistance, release your pressure at the very beginning of inhalation. However, our impression is that this has more effect on the sternochondral joints than on the lung itself.

Treatment of the *right oblique fissural region* is similar, but with the patient in left lateral decubitus position. Both these techniques can be performed with one hand stretching the right arm while the treating hand pushes on the ribs.

For a *double pressure technique,* put the patient in supine position, stand behind his head, and place both palms against the anterolateral parts of ribs 5 and 6. Press your

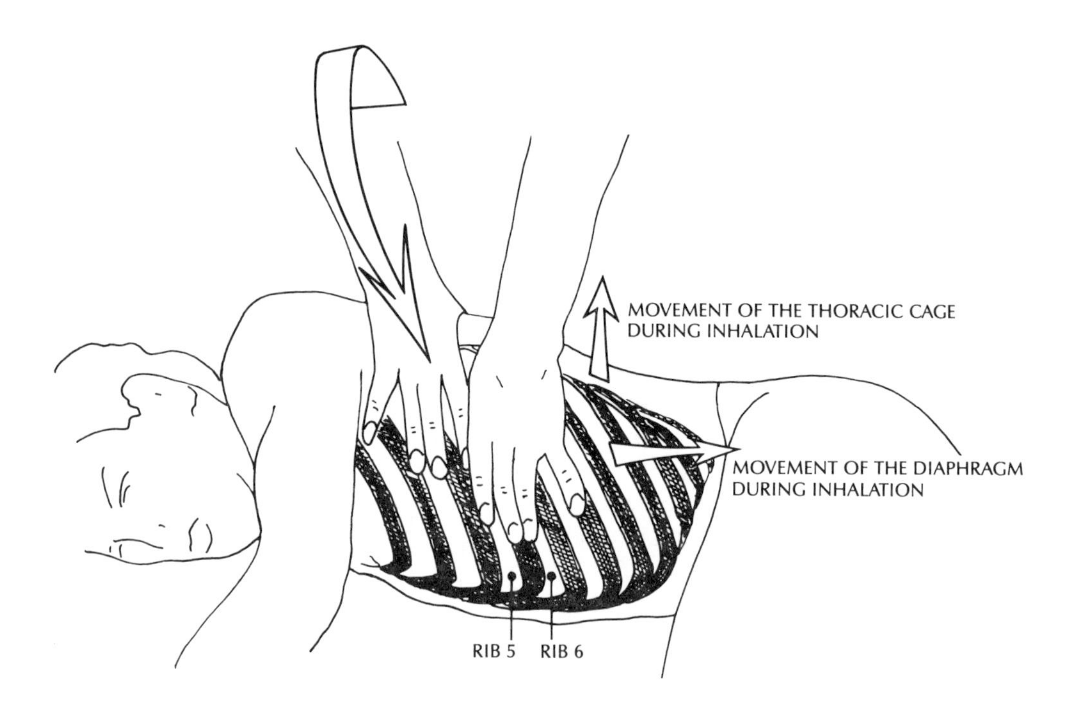

Illustration 6-16
Release of the Left Horizontal Fissural Region

hands toward each other. Maintain this compression at the end of exhalation and then ask the patient to inhale slowly and deeply to induce stretching. For recoil with respiratory assistance, let go at the very beginning of inhalation.

HEART

In the early stages of our practice, we treated many patients who had undergone open heart surgery. They were not suffering from actual cardiac pain, but the thorax was traumatized from the operation. Later, we treated more patients with coronary artery disease in whom listening tests and manual thermal diagnosis showed up the restrictions well. During listening, our hands were invariably drawn toward the coronary arteries. We carried out stretching movements along the orientation of the arteries, and the patients usually reported significant relief. The technique is described below. We must caution you to talk to the patient in terms of "thoracic stretching" rather than "coronary stretching," since we have no evidence that this technique actually affects these arteries. We know only that it brings relief. Before applying these techniques to a patient with established coronary artery disease, be certain that there are no signs of an infarct.

Place the patient in supine position, hands on his abdomen. Stand behind the patient's head, cross your arms, and place your right hand on the third left sternochondral joint, the left between the third and fourth right sternochondrals. Push both hands posterolaterally and inferiorly, with an amount of force similar to that used for stretching a rib. Push during exhalation when the thorax is less rigid. On the right the direction of force is at 40 degrees from the midline; on the left there is much less lateral force, at 20 degrees from the midline (Illustration 6-17).

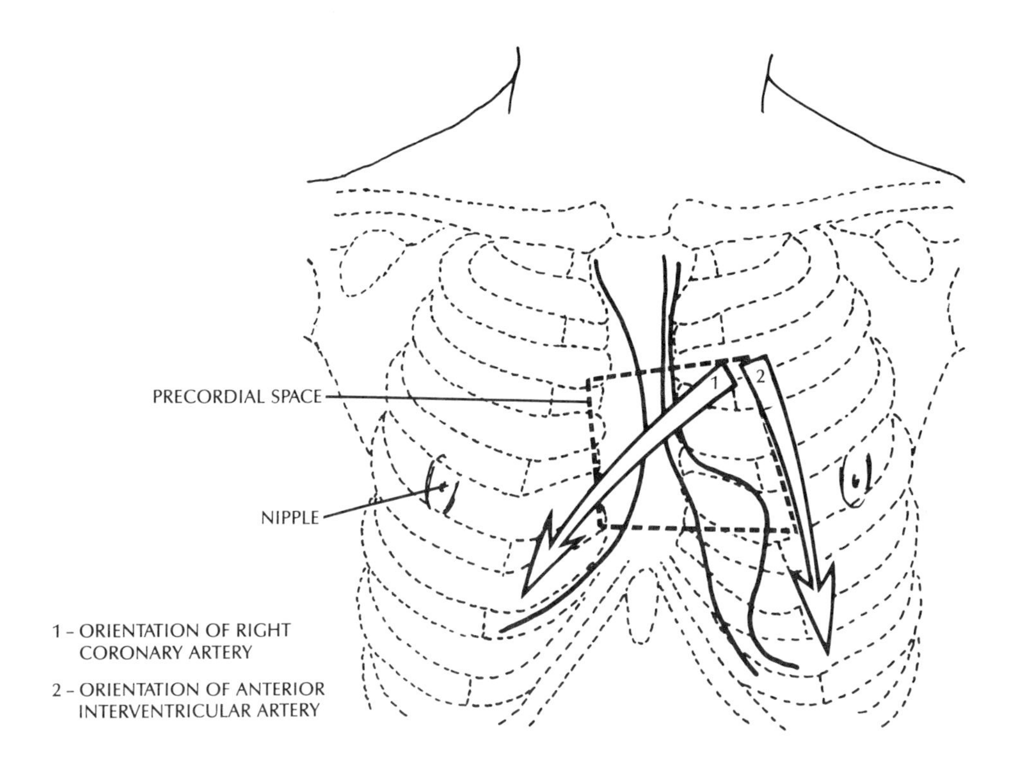

Illustration 6-17
Stretching along the Orientation of the Coronary Arteries

By working on only one direction at a time you can be more focused and precise. Initially, the other hand is just used for stabilization. As you proceed it gently pushes laterally toward the opposite side, which aids in the stretching. For example, when you stretch along the orientation of the left coronary artery your right hand pushes in the direction of that artery; the left hand is on the third left sternochondral joint and pushes to the right in order to increase the stretching effect. As the technique continues, your hands move progressively farther. Treatment is complete when no further movement is possible and no more changes are felt in the ribs or soft tissues.

Nerves and Plexuses

Effects of manipulation on nervous system structures can be quite dramatic. We will restrict our discussion here to the phrenic nerve and the three most important plexuses affecting thoracic function.

PHRENIC NERVE

Place your thumb in the access point for the phrenic nerve (see Illustration 5-5). On listening, you will feel a slight sliding motion going alternately superior-inferior, medial-lateral, or anterior-posterior. This is different from the clockwise-counterclockwise rotation of the plexuses. Stimulating the phrenic nerve has a beneficial effect on the motions of the thoracic organs, and helps release the diaphragm. To do this, slightly exaggerate the speed and amplitude of the motion you feel on listening until you feel a release and the motion stops. With emotionally-related disorders of the thorax or diaphragm, it is helpful to treat the phrenic nerve bilaterally. To further release the diaphragm, it is a good idea to simultaneously inhibit the access point of the phrenic nerve and de Mussy's point.

PLEXUSES

The plexuses are released by going in the direction of listening, returning to the original position, and repeating this until the movement stops by itself (see *Visceral Manipulation II*, p. 30). For treatment of the *celiac plexus*, put the patient in supine position, arms and legs stretched out, and stand to one side. Place one palm on the upper abdomen, the thenar or hypothenar eminence against the seventh right costochondral joint and the rest of the hand pointing toward the midline. Pressure of the hand should be light to avoid feeling the motility of the adjacent organs.

Treatment of the *superficial cardiac plexus* is similar, except that you place your hand on the third and fourth left sternochondral cartilages, the middle finger making a 30 degree angle with the midline.

For treatment of the *stellate ganglion*, the patient can be in either seated or supine position. With the seated position, sit behind the patient with one hand resting on his sternoclavicular junction, its thumb over the surface projection of the ganglion. This is the anterior part of the transverse process of C7. In overweight patients this is nearly impossible to find, so your thumb is placed near the anterolateral part of the first costovertebral joint. When the patient is supine, place the thenar eminence of your hand on the sternum and the index or middle finger over the ganglion. Listening to the ganglion brings the finger or thumb into slight clockwise and counterclockwise axial rotation, with some medial-lateral sliding. The palm of the sternal hand moves little or not at all. You should always treat the stellate ganglion bilaterally. However, treatment of the right ganglion is more effective than that of the left, for reasons we do not understand. The pressure applied by your thumb or finger must be moderate. If it causes discomfort, coughing, or miosis of the ipsilateral eye, you are pressing too hard.

COORDINATION OF THE PLEXUSES

It is important that the plexuses not only each function well individually, but that they also be coordinated with each other (this is similar to the sphincter-like areas). For thoracic problems we are accustomed to coordinating the celiac and cardiac plexuses with each other, followed by the stellate ganglion. Your goal is to give the plexuses a listening movement of the same rhythm and amplitude, which will cause movement in both to diminish and eventually stop completely. When you are treating two plexuses at the same time, your body should be equidistant from them, and you must concentrate equally on both. After doing this you will either feel no motion (which signifies successful release of both plexuses), or motion resumes in both (which means you have to continue).

For example, if you want to release the cardiac plexus, you first treat it by itself. You then coordinate it with the celiac plexus, and next with the stellate ganglion. Finally, you confirm your results by comparing the stellate ganglion and celiac plexus. If you are repeatedly unsuccessful with this approach, you will need to use the left frontal lobe to aid in the coordination. Leave one hand on the plexus that has the greatest amplitude of listening motion, place the other on the left frontal, and continue with your attempt at coordination.

Based on our clinical experience, we believe that the left frontal is the location (or at least the surface projection) of the individual's emotions, social and familial relationships, personality, etc. It is your face to other people. The right frontal is your very deep self, your fundamental character, your face to yourself. We call the left frontal the "commander-in-chief" of the plexuses because information from the plexuses (on social stresses, etc.) is directed here for integration. The right frontal only becomes involved when the problem is too large or demanding for the left frontal to handle. For coordination of the left frontal, place your hand on the left forehead and proceed as for a plexus.

Coordination of the plexuses, as briefly described here, is the beginning of visceroemotional treatment, which involves the use of specific organs to arouse or diminish emotions in the mind. Understanding these techniques and presenting them in detail is our primary project for the next few years.

Advice

Our general strategy for treatment is to release in the following order:

- muscular and fascial systems,
- visceral system,
- osteoarticular system,
- plexuses (including coordination).

We tend to avoid specific adjustment techniques, particularly for the vertebrae. Such techniques can certainly be very effective, but they often hide and short-circuit other imbalances in the tissues. We therefore begin with techniques to release muscles, fasciae, and viscera. In this way, through gradual loosening of the soft tissues, the significant osteoarticular restrictions become obvious. There are some exceptions. For example, you need to release the subclavius muscle and corresponding conoid and trapezoid ligaments before treating a restricted middle cervical aponeurosis. Before and after each treatment, check Adson-Wright test results and arterial pressure of both arms. These can serve as useful reference points for evaluation of your success.

Sometimes you will be surprised by the pathological effect of some minor restriction, one which may strike you as irrelevant. For example, release of a small sternochondral restriction can have a far-reaching positive effect on thoracic function and efficiency of respiration. Diagnosis of these small restrictions is difficult, and you will need to be familiar with a variety of mobility tests and local and general listening tests. For this purpose, we urge you to review the techniques described in our previous books.

While this book is finished, we know that all we have done is to push the door to inquiry ajar. It is our hope that we will all continue to research the intrathoracic system using our long-standing principles:

- continually study anatomy using books, imaging techniques, and dissections;
- base our work firmly on clinical practice;
- try to let all the body's messages pass through our hands, which have to both feel and treat at the same time; and
- link the body to the mind.

Bibliography

Barral, J-P. *Visceral Manipulation II.* Seattle: Eastland Press, 1989.

Barral, J-P., Mathieu, J-P., Mercier, P. *Diagnostic articulaire vertébral.* Charleroir: S.B.O.R.T.M., 1981.

Barral, J-P., Mercier, P. *Visceral Manipulation.* Seattle: Eastland Press, 1988.

Bochuberg, C. *Traitement ostéopathique des rhinites et sinusites chroniques.* Paris: Maloine, 1986.

Braunwald, E. et. al., eds. *Harrison's Principles of Internal Medicine.* NY: McGraw-Hill, 1987.

Chauffour, P., Guillot, J-M. *Le Lien mécanique ostéopathique.* Paris: Maloine, 1985.

Comroe, J.H. *Physiologie de la respiration.* Paris: Masson, 1978.

Contamin, R.; Bernard, P. *Gynécolgie générale.* Paris: Vigot, 1977.

Cruveilhier, J. *Traité d'anatomie humaine.* Paris: Octave Doin, 1852.

Davenport, H.W. *Physiologie de l'appareil digestif.* Paris: Masson, 1976.

Delmas, A. *Vies et Centres Nerveux.* Paris: Masson, 1975.

Dousset, H. *L'examen du malade en clientèle.* Paris: Maloine, 1972.

Gararel, B.; Roques, M. *Les fasciae.* Paris: Maloine, 1985.

Grégoire, R.; Oberlin, S. *Précis d'anatomie.* Paris: J.P. Ballière, 1973.

Herman, J.; Cier, J.F. *Précis de physiologie.* Paris: Masson, 1977.

Hughes, F. Cl. *Pathologie respiratoire.* Paris: Heures de France, 1971.

Issarter, L. & M. *L'Ostéopathie exactement.* Paris: Robert Laffont, 1983.

Kahle, W.; Leonhardt, H.; Platzer, W. *Anatomie des viscères.* Paris: Flammarion, 1978.

Kamina, P. *Anatomie gynécologique obstrétricale.* Paris: Maloine, 1984.

Korr, I. *The Neurobiologic Mechanisms in Manipulative Therapy.* NY: Plenum, 1978.

Laborit, H. *L'Inhibition de l'action. Biologie, physiologie, psychologie, sociologie.* Paris: Maddon, 1981.

Lansac, J.; Lecomte, P. *Gynécologie pour le praticien.* Villeurbanne: Simep, 1981.

Lavielle, J.; Roux, J.; Stanoyevitch, J-F.. *Le système vertébro-basilaire.* Marseille, 1981.

Lazorthes, G. *Le système nerveux périphérique.* Paris, Masson, 1971.

Poirier, P.; Charpy, A.; Nicolas, A. *Taité d'anatomie humaine* (Tomes I-V). Paris: Masson, 1912.

Prefaut, C. *L'essentiel en physiologie respiratoire.* Paris: Sauramps Médical, 1986.

Renaud, R., et.al., *Les incontinences urinaires chez la femme.* Paris: Masson, 1982.

Robert, J.G., et.al., *Précis de gynécologie.* Paris: Masson, 1974.

Rouvier, H. *Anatomie humaine.* Paris: Masson, 1967.

Scali, P., Warrel, D. W. *Les prolapsus vaginaux et l'incontinence urinaires chex la femme.* Paris, Masson, 1980.

Taurelle, R. *Obstetrique.* Paris: France Médical Edition, 1980.

Testut, L. *Traité d'anatomie humaine.* Paris: Gaston Doin, 1889

Testus, L., Jacob, O. *Anatomie topographique.* Paris: Gaston Doin, 1889.

de Tourris, H., Henrion, R., Delecour, M. *Gynécologie et obstrétrique.* Paris: Masson, 1979.

Upledger, J.E., Vredevoogd, J.D. *Craniosacral Therapy.* Seattle: Eastland Press, 1983.

Waligora, H., Perlemuter, L. *Anatomie.* Paris: Masson, 1975.

West, J.B. *Physiologie respiratoire.* Paris: Medsi, 1986.

Wright, S. *Physiologie appliquée à la médecine.* Paris: Flammarion, 1974.

Williams, P.; Warwick, R, eds. *Gray's Anatomy.* Edinburgh: Livingstone, 1980.

List of Illustrations

CHAPTER TWO

CHAPTER THREE

CHAPTER FIVE

CHAPTER SIX

Index

Numbers in boldface refer to an illustration.